THE WELLNESS CODE

Your Ultimate Guide to **Health, Fitness & Nutrition**

Published by CelebrityPress™, Orlando, FL
A division of The Celebrity Branding Agency®

Celebrity Branding® is a registered trademark
Printed in the United States of America.

ISBN: 9780983947059
LCCN: 2011945054

For more information, please write:

CelebrityPress™,

520 N. Orlando Ave, #2
Winter Park, FL 32789
or call 1.877.261.4930

Visit us online at www.CelebrityPressPublishing.com

THE WELLNESS CODE

Your Ultimate Guide to **Health, Fitness & Nutrition**

Contents

FOREWORD

By Kelli Calabrese 15

CHAPTER 1

THE BIG PICTURE OF WELLNESS - ACTIONS AND MINDSET

By John Spencer Ellis, EdD 19

CHAPTER 2

YOUR WISH IS MY COMMAND…

By Linda M. McCarthy, Ph.D 29

CHAPTER 3

BAD HABITS BE GONE

By Mallory Cargile 39

CHAPTER 4

MASTERING YOUR BODY

By Briar Munro 49

CHAPTER 5

THE ART OF BREATHING
REDUCE STRESS AND TENSION
IN LESS THAN 10 MINUTES PER DAY

By Lisa Fox Bail, CK 59

CHAPTER 6

DANDELION DREAMS

By La-Verne Parris 69

CHAPTER 7

HOW TO BE SUCCESSFUL AND STILL HAVE A LIFE!

By Helen M. Thamm, MS, APRN, CPC 79

CHAPTER 8

THE BEST ANTI-AGING SECRET EVER

By Annie Hodgskiss 87

CHAPTER 9

FIVE STEPS TO PEAK PERFORMANCE IN SPORTS

By Gavin Kent 99

CHAPTER 10

EIGHT TIPS TO HELP YOU IMPROVE AND KEEP YOUR NUTRITIONAL HABITS

By Dexter Tenison 105

CHAPTER 11

7 STEPS TO THRIVE

By Camille Scielzi 113

CHAPTER 12

TWO BLOOD TESTS THAT CAN SAVE YOUR LIFE

By Inger Pols 123

CHAPTER 13

DISCOVERING HEALTH THROUGH ADVERSITY

By Sabreena CopeLyn, PhD, ACPEC, SPHR 133

CHAPTER 14

FACING LIFE'S CHALLENGES – A HOLISTIC PERSPECTIVE

By Lisa Mercier 143

CHAPTER 15

LIFESTYLE ENHANCEMENT – MIND AND MEDITATION

FOR STRESS, PAIN, SLEEP, MEMORY, TIME MANAGEMENT, PRODUCTIVITY, HAPPINESS, AND MORE

By Katrina Luise Everhart, RYT 153

CHAPTER 16

TRUTH OR DARE

By Warren Martin 163

CHAPTER 17

YOUR PERSONAL 30-DAY WELLNESS CODE

By David Krainiak 173

CHAPTER 18

GET YOUR GLOW ON!

RADIANT HEALTHY SKIN STARTS FROM THE INSIDE OUT

By Diane Scarazzini.. 183

CHAPTER 19

THE FIT MOM MINDSET

By Joe Martin 195

CHAPTER 20

BALANCE – THE SECRET TO LASTING FITNESS

By Michael Coleman 203

CHAPTER 21

CREATE YOUR OWN EXTREME BODY/LIFE MAKEOVER

By Kevin M. Harvey & Kristen Harvey DPT 213

CHAPTER 22

UNLOCKING THE CODE

By Gregg Viscuso 223

CHAPTER 23

CHANGE YOUR LIFESTYLE, CHANGE YOUR LIFE

10 SIMPLE STEPS TO A HAPPY, HEALTHY YOU!

Justine SanFilippo 235

CHAPTER 24

FLEX YOUR JOY

By Dorothy Jantzen 245

CHAPTER 25

THE NEW WARRIOR BLUEPRINT FOR HEALTH & LONGEVITY

By Sincere Hogan 255

CHAPTER 26

CREATING A ROAD MAP TO HEALTH, WELLNESS AND BALANCE

By Doug Duerr 265

CHAPTER 27

OCCUPATIONAL WELLNESS!

By Raymond James 277

Foreword

By Kelli Calabrese

For the first time in history, lifestyle diseases like diabetes, heart disease, and cancer kill more people than communicable disease. You can't help but stop and ask yourself what are we doing so dramatically wrong in our lifestyles to be in such a state of dis-ease. While the world is advancing technologically, more people are living in bodies that are burdened with being un-well.

In the 1970's, 1-in-12 people in the United States had cancer. In the 1990's, it jumped drastically to 1-in-4. Today, statistically, every other person will be plagued with cancer. Add to that the grueling facts that 74.6% of Americans are obese or overweight, 90% of heart disease is lifestyle-related, and it costs trillions of dollars to treat these conditions. These problems are debilitating and often fatal to the people who suffer with them.

The great news is… ***it does not have to be that way!*** We are living during the best times in all of history and our potential for enjoying great physical health is unlimited.

A study of nearly 45,000 sets of twins in 2000 found that environment factors and lifestyle habits were stronger predictors than genetic factors – when determining who will get sick or be well, regarding lifestyle diseases. So your choices do matter!

This means that everyone can walk in health, even in ultra-health! Diseases of civilization are preventable, and they are prevented the same way they are caused – lifestyle! A wholesome diet, regular exercise, sweet sleep, life ownership, a spiritual connection and detoxification are possible for each and every one of us.

I always say, "Show me one." If one person can quit smoking, you can too. If a new mom can get her body back and better, so can you. If a post-menopausal woman can enjoy seven solid hours of sleep and a sexy body, there is hope for you. If a couch potato can grace the stage of a body-building contest, there's promise for all of us.

The hope lies in three components:
First, you need a belief that positive change is possible. You must have faith that there is potential for even you, no matter where you sit as you read this. No matter how far gone you may think you are, or even if you are simply trying to fine-tune a few elements of your well-being, your mind must be in agreement with forward progress. The mind is a powerful tool, and if you approach change with positivity, your actions will follow your thoughts. Make up your mind and set your sights on the best possible health achievable for you!

Second, you must possess sound, practical and proven principles to achieve wellness. That's where this book has fallen into your hands as *the* solution! It's no accident that *The Wellness Code* has worked its way into your life at this very time. This book was compiled from the minds of the most talented 'wellness experts.' They have included the latest information combined with the best practical tools they have had consistent success with – coaching their numerous clients.

Finally, you need to follow through. You need to show up for your workouts, plan ahead for solid sleep, make the best possible food choices, manage your stress, keep toxins at bay and maintain a spiritual walk. It's all laid out for you in the Wellness Code! It's possible. There are many people who are enjoying walking in optimal health and you can too – within a short period of time of making the decision to turn the next page.

Right now, you have habits that have been ingrained over time. You have habits about exercising, or lack thereof. You already have a breakfast habit – even if that means you skip it or have dessert for breakfast. You have sleeping habits and eating habits. One step at a time, improvements can and will be made to every area of your life as you move forward.

Now is the perfect time to ask yourself how satisfied you are with your energy, the amount of over-the-counter or prescription medication you are taking, the health of your family, the results you are having from your exercise program, your waist line and the direction your health is headed. Are you finishing up this year healthier than you started? That's not the case for most. You can be the exception.

I'm going to bet that if you picked up a copy of *The Wellness Code*, you want more. You want to crack the code to living in natural health, to feeling your best and looking fantastic at any age. The information you are about to read has the potential to be the most influential health-enhancing knowledge you need to finally achieve the wellness goals you desire.

I encourage you to not only read the words, but let them sink into your mind, and then apply them wholeheartedly. A short time from now you will notice a boost to your energy, then better-fitting clothing, then some more definition in your muscles, followed by the reduction and even elimination of medication, managed stress and much more. I've even had clients tell me they are happier after applying the principles in *The Wellness Code.*

I invite you to be well. You deserve it. Wellness awaits on the pages that lie ahead. Extraordinary health will be yours!

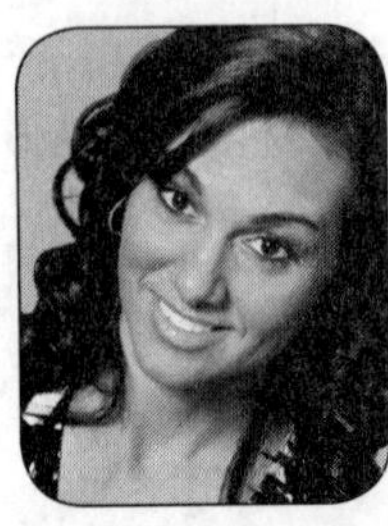

Kelli Calabrese

Kelli is a Clinical Exercise Physiologist. She has been a fitness, nutrition and wellness leader for the past 25 years. Kelli was the lead fitness expert for eDiets & eFitness. She is the fitness expert for Montel Williams and is the international master trainer for Adventure Boot Camp. Kelli is the author of *Feminine, Firm & Fit*, a consultant with Isagenix and a Founder of Beyond Organics. She is an international presenter on topics including metabolism and detoxification, and is also a keynote speaker for Fortune 500 companies. She has owned and operated fitness centers and managed many corporate fitness facilities.

Kelli is a native New Yorker and resides in the Dallas area with her husband of almost 20 years and her two amazing children, Nicholas and Melina.

For more information:
www.KelliCalabrese.com
Kelli@KelliCalabrese.com

CHAPTER 1

The Big Picture of Wellness - Actions and Mindset

By John Spencer Ellis, EdD

The Wellness Code is packed full of golden nuggets of wisdom to help you live a life of enhanced wellness and abundant health. But, what does that mean? Is wellness a group of ideas, concepts and practices, or something much more?

In this chapter you will learn more about the overarching theme of wellness, and why it can just be a group of ideas, concepts and practices. In that case, you will experience enhanced wellness. However, when you embrace being a "well person," everything seems to fall into place, and the result is a new, rebuilt and completely whole YOU.

I think a definition is in order. Yes, we all have a slightly different take on wellness, but I think my co-authors will fundamentally agree with me here. Wellness can be defined as the collective rituals, behaviors, practices and lifestyle traits that lead to better health, improved sleep, faster recovery, increased happiness and better social experiences.

We all slice the "wellness pie" (often called a Wellness Wheel) a little differently. I think all perspectives have merit. The basic premise is learning what slices are needed to make a whole pie. The fact that we use a pie of any kind for a pictorial representation of wellness is a bit ironic. One of the first things you must do is decide what ingredients will make up your pie. Yes, there are a few fundamentals such as sleep, exercise and nutrition, which should be included in each model.

Now is the time for you to really think this through. What does wellness mean to you? If you are a single person, does surrounding yourself with friends fill the possible void of not having an immediate family? How would your "social" piece of pie be as compared to other slices? Do all pieces of your pie have to be symmetrical? This would be an indicator that you are in a need of balance: How is your pie sliced compared to that of other people close to you? It's okay, and even good, to be different.

I'm going to throw a wrench in this whole wellness thing right now. I'm going to propose you don't need, or even want, balance as it is often prescribed. Wow. Bold statement. Before you go off and tell people I'm nuts, just think of this for a moment. Nothing is in perfect balance. Nothing. There is always a counter movement, an adjustment, a counter weight, or a tweak of some kind. In short, feel free to have a lumpy pie.

Here are some examples of what I mean: Some people do well with seven hours of sleep, while others need nine to function properly. Some individuals achieve all of their fitness goals with just 30 minutes of exercise a day, while others cannot imagine doing less than 90 minutes on most days. Men can frequently eat far more than women without adding unwanted body fat. Some people indulge in various spiritual or religious practices on a daily basis as a regular practice to keep themselves grounded, while others get spiritual enrichment going to a soup kitchen and feeding the homeless once a week. In short, we are all unique. As you develop your wellness pie, make sure you are doing so on your terms, with your specific values and goals in mind.

OBJECTIVES, STRATEGIES AND TACTICS

These are powerful words: objectives, strategies and tactics. They are most often reserved for defining business success principles. Let's discuss how they equally apply to your wellness journey.

- An **objective** is something worked toward or striven for—a goal.
- A **strategy** is a plan of action intended to accomplish a specific goal.
- A **tactic** is a procedure or set of maneuvers engaged in to achieve an end, an aim, or a goal.

Now the application:

What is your overall objective with your wellness plan? Do you want to live longer? Do you want to increase your energy? Do you want to improve your physical appearance?

You have to know your desired outcome so you will know how to delegate your time, money and effort (investment) in your wellness program.

There is something I need to mention right here and now. Your daily activities and actions must be congruent with your overall objective. EXAMPLE: You cannot have a primary goal of youthful energy and appearance if you never include sleep science and skin treatments in your regime. Makes sense, right? Stay focused on your objective.

The strategies you use for wellness give you more creative freedom and require more thought. EXAMPLES: If your objective is to run a marathon, a strategy is to hire a running coach. If your objective is to improve your eating habits and learn about the best foods for your overall objective and personal taste, you should hire a dietitian as a strategy.

The tactics are the details. They are the specifics of your strategies and the minutiae of your objective. EXAMPLES: Your objective is to improve overall endurance. Your strategies include riding your bike in a 100-mile charity event, and hiring a cycling coach to ensure success. The tactics you will use to ensure that your strategies and objectives are successful can include the following: taking specific shorter rides leading to longer rides, getting a custom bike fit, buying snacks for longer training rides, and getting a massage before the big event.

Take a moment right now and think about your overall objective with your wellness plan. Make sure your daily activities and actions are congruent with your overall objective. What strategies are needed? What tactics will you use? To me, this is actually the fun part. You will be better prepared and enjoy much better results. It's important to note that there will most likely be adjustments, modifications, and deletions as your wellness plan comes into shape. It's to be expected. It's normal. Adjust and move on.

LET'S TALK ABOUT YOUR MIND.

One of the coolest things I've ever heard said about the mind is this: If our brain was so simple we could understand it, we would be so simple we couldn't. If that wasn't cool enough, how about this: If you believe we only use 10% of our brain, then you would also have to believe that if you learn 90% more, you are done learning.

What does all this mean?

I'll get right to the point and then give you the details. Your wellness is only as strong, as good, and as long-lasting as your mind is powerful. Is this gobbledygook? No. This is scientific fact and the premise of all successful endeavors in life.

Think of the Olympic athlete with incredible focus. Imagine the monk who can control his breathing and body temperature, and can ignore extreme temperatures. Picture the almost zen-like state of an archer who puts her sights on the target. This is the focus that is ideal for the ultimate results in your wellness plan.

At this point, you may be thinking that this is too much work! Well, it doesn't have to be that way. It's more of a method of approaching life. This is where we really get into what I originally said, "Embrace being a well person." This is a whole paradigm shift.

YOU ARE NOW A WELL PERSON.

So, when you wake up in the morning, you now have an entirely new perspective of life and how you live it. You live it the "wellness way." It starts with how you approach the first few moments of the day. Seriously, it matters. Decide your day will be fun, invigorating and productive. Create a morning ritual for success. Gently shake your arms and legs, take some deep, full breaths and do your morning necessities.

Within 10 - 15 minutes, drink some water. You get dehydrated overnight and your brain will function better if you are well hydrated. When possible (everyone's schedule is different), exercise in the morning. Studies show people are far more committed to morning exercise routines as compared to the evening. Other benefits include increased metabolism throughout the day, better sleep patterns, and a sense of accomplishment to move you forward for the rest of the day.

Everyone's wellness pie has a slice for work or contribution. So, we must include it here as well. As you go through your work day, focus on productivity and task completion, rather than just being busy. Avoid the *bright shiny object syndrome* that afflicts most people. In other words, do not allow remedial tasks and frivolous invasions of your time to remove you from the highest levels of productivity and accomplishment. Yes, having a greater sense of purpose and accomplishment will improve your wellness.

Every decision has benefits and consequences. Yes, that may sound really serious when we're talking about wellness, so let me explain. As you go about your day, each choice you make will have an impact on your health and wellness. However, now that you are a well person, you look at things differently. This does not mean that you increase stress worrying about every little imaginable aspect of your daily rituals, wondering if it was the best possible move for optimal wellness. That would be counter productive. Think of it as more of a simple check and balance sheet. It has give and take, ebb and flow. If you decide to have a high-sugar cereal, you should not feel guilty. Instead, you would ask yourself questions such as, "Am I feeling low in energy this morning and only think I need sugar?" or "Am I using this as a means of rewarding myself for something. If so, what is a better choice?"

Something that I have done for years, and one I'm going to invite you to try is this: If I eat something that is a poor choice, I know the same day I will do a bit more cardio, drink an extra glass of water, and remember to take my vitamins. I don't freak out, get depressed, or feel guilty. That never works well over time. Just realize that you need to take some positive countermeasures. Move on.

Part of your daily wellness ritual is to take time. Take time to rest. Take time to reflect. Take time to dream. Take time to plan. Some of the best advice I ever received was from my yoga master, Erich Schiffmann. He is a yoga legend, and learning from him was life altering. His philosophy is about "Moving into Stillness." He says, "Be in the now." Stillness doesn't just happen. It's more of a transition, a transcendence. I don't want to get woo-woo here. Just think about it. Relaxation is a process. There are levels. It takes time. It's a learned behavior and practice.

EATING

You need to take time when transitioning from an active part of your day to meal time. You need to redirect your thoughts and your blood flow to your digestion. This, along with being thankful for your food, improves digestion. This is what is known as food psychology. Marc David is the pioneer of this work. Each time I sit down to eat, as hungry as I may be, I take 10 - 20 deep breaths before I take my first bite. I also let go of whatever may be on my mind (work, training, challenges) and focus on the food. When eating, make sure you get vitamin T and vitamin O. Vitamin T is time. Take your time when you eat. You will eat less, feel better, and improve your health. Vitamin O is oxygen. Continue to take deep breaths while you are eating. Increasing oxygen intake while eating improves digestion. Yes, this may be simple, but I bet you do not do this at every meal. It works.

Take time to daydream. It happened all the time when you were a kid. Then at some point, it slowed to a crawl, and sometimes it completely stops. Wow. That is not good. You now have permission to daydream. It feels good. It reduces stress. It's what leads to better choices. It helps shape your future, and custom design your life. Consider taking a walk and do what is called *active meditation*. Essentially, that means you are not sitting down with your legs crossed. Choose a safe, quiet place where you can take an easy stroll and focus your thoughts, or let it all go. This is great practice 15 minutes following a meal. It can help digestion.

Take time to assess and take inventory. In one of your 10-minute timeouts, take an inventory of your day. Ask yourself the following: How do I feel? How is my energy? Do I have a sense of accomplishment? What is my happiness level? What excites me? What excites me about tomorrow? It's important to be in the now, and be excited about tomorrow, too.

EXERCISE

As mentioned earlier, exercising in the morning is advised. Regardless of when you exercise, there are some fundamentals to remember, regardless of your personal goals.

First, respect your body. You have to be honest with yourself about what is possible and for what reasons you are on a particular fitness quest. As you hone your wellness skills, your ability to self-assess will improve. Become acutely aware of aches and pains. Learn to differentiate between the good and bad pain. Learn to detect body imbalances. By this I mean structural imbalances. Is one shoulder higher than the other? Does it feel like your pelvis is rotated? Is one side of your body dramatically less flexible or weaker than the other side? Some slight imbalances are to be expected. But a major imbalance could lead to early arthritis, significant soft tissue damage, decreased sports performance and pain. If you detect these imbalances, I suggest seeing a chiropractor and corrective exercise specialist.

Avoid overtraining. If you are questioning whether you are doing too much, you likely are. If you cannot recover from a workout in 48 hours, you are probably overdoing it. When in doubt about your training program, seek the advice of an expert. You will enjoy better results, fewer injuries, and you will reach your goals more quickly.

SLEEP

Oh, how beautiful is sleep? It is quite possibly my favorite part of the day. I invite you to think about sleep differently beginning right now. Sleep is also a transition. When you close your eyes, you are removing yourself from the day and embracing the night. As with your midday breaks, it's a process. At night, you don't just lay your head down and are fast asleep. In fact, if that is the case, you are overtired. It should take about 10-15 minutes to "release" the day and gently go to sleep.

I'd like to give you some specific information to help you get a better night's sleep. Sleep is good! Your body's core temperature lowers at night. An optimal temperature for sleep is 65 degrees Fahrenheit with 65% humidity. As you prepare for bed, have a ritual. This ritual reminds your body that it's time to let go and allow any stress and worries from the day to subside. Rituals are personal and can include meditation, a bath, gentle stretching, deep breathing or listening to relaxing music. Make your bedroom as dark as possible. A darker room allows for better melatonin secretions and this deepens your sleep. Remove as many electronics from your room as possible. You don't need the distraction, light or electronic fields. Here's an interesting tidbit—stay off your cell phone for the 30 minutes prior to sleep.

Some studies show that the cell phone can reduce melatonin secretion.

So there you have it. You now know the primary physical and mental skills to enhance your wellness. **You have gone from a person who wants to be well to a well person.**

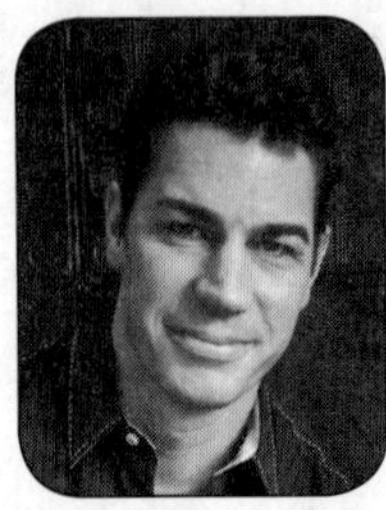

About John

Each week, over one million people enjoy a fitness, wellness and personal success program created by John Spencer Ellis. His programs are implemented in the top resorts, spas and fitness centers. John is the CEO of the National Exercise & Sports Trainers Association (NESTA), Spencer Institute for Life Coaching, International Triathlon Coaching Association (ITCA), and the Mixed Martial Arts Conditioning Association (MMACA).

John created Adventure Boot Camp, the largest fitness boot camp system in the world. He also created Intense Mixed Performance Accelerated Cross Training (IMPACT), Kung-fu Fitness and TACTIX. His TriActive America signature series of outdoor exercise equipment is used worldwide. He created programs used by Cirque du Soleil, the U.S. Secret Service, Army, Navy, Air Force, Marines and Coast Guard, and consults the UFC (Ultimate Fighting Championships).

John holds two bachelor's degrees (business & health science), an MBA, and a doctorate in education. He also completed doctoral level studies in naturopathic health education. He holds fifteen certifications in health and fitness. John has ridden his bicycle enough miles to circle the Earth. He raced in cycling and triathlon competitions for over 10 years. He completed the Ironman triathlon and finished 5th at the U.S. National Biathlon Championships. John holds a 2nd degree black belt in Kung-fu, and a black belt in Ninjutsu. He now trains in Krav Maga, Brazilian Jiu Jitsu, and Kempo Karate. He has experience in Muay Thai and boxing.

John is a certified instructor of self-defense, fitness kick boxing and fitness boxing. He was nominated for the California Community College Distinguished Alumni Award and nominated for induction into the Fitness Hall of Fame.

For detailed information and great FREE GIFTS, visit:
www.johnspencerellis.com

CHAPTER 2

Your Wish Is My Command...

By Linda M. McCarthy, Ph.D

Can negative thoughts, feelings and emotions play a significant role in our physiology, or are they just words that have no genuine importance? Let's take a look at the meaning of the word **'emotion'** in the dictionary.

The word emotion is derived from the Latin term *'emotus'* or *'emovere'*: to move outward. When the ability to skillfully channel emotions are developed, this enables us to move effortlessly through life with little discord. However, what if a person is not proficient in understanding the possible consequences of continual pessimism? At what point does a negative emotion become so toxic to the body that it begins to affect overall health?

Until I began my journey to understand the mind-body connection, I had a limited understanding between the direct correlation of a negative thought or emotion, and the physiological response that occurred in the body at that moment. I grew up overhearing others complain about a situation or person causing them to experience: *"A pain in their neck"*; *"a thorn in their side"*; or feeling *"broken hearted."* These comments were metaphoric expressions of course, but they also represented a reflection of an actual physical sensation. I assumed they were just common terminologies used to convey emotional discomfort. After all, how could a thought or a feeling affect our physical health? They were only fleeting aphorisms and we could change them at will, or could we?

Basically there are two types of thoughts, supportive and non-supportive. Your self-concept is based on how you speak to yourself, consciously and subconsciously. I often convey to clients: *"Be careful what you are thinking, your cells are listening,"* because in a sense the receptors on the cells act as antennas or ears, and they are vibrationally eavesdropping on our thoughts. When we find ourselves in a toxic environment, or experience negativity for extended periods of time, on a conscious level we convince ourselves that all is well, and the situation is under control. However subconsciously, if we do not believe what we are thinking, our cells will respond accordingly. If the belief continues for an extended period of time, the cells and the DNA will adapt and change according to their environment. These changes eventually manifest into physical and mental dis-ease in the body. As signals are sent from the environment, positive or negative, the cells respond in like. I compare the cellular response in our body to a genie in a bottle: *"Your wish is my command."* I would like to share a very personal story in which this theory applies.

A very close friend of mine Laurel, was diagnosed with pancreatic cancer a few years ago. She was informed by the medical community that her tumor was too large, discovered too late, and regrettably, there was nothing they could do for her. She was told to go home, get her affairs in order, call Hospice, and make any other arrangements necessary for her inevitable demise. Fortunately, Laurel LOVED life, so she relentless pursed doctor after doctor until she found one who agreed to administer chemotherapy and radiation in an attempt to shrink the size of the tumor, thus allowing for its removal in surgery. In the meantime, Laurel continued to enjoy her wonderful life, even purchasing a brand new sports car in anticipation of the surgery which had yet to be scheduled.

She expected a positive outcome and was excited to drive the car that awaited her after recovery. Believing the physician's protocol would work since the tumor had shrunk significantly, Laurel had the surgery and the operation was a complete success. She was cancer free and even complied with the physician's request for additional chemotherapy treatments to ensure total elimination of any rogue malignant cells. What puzzled both Laurel and I was that she always appeared to be optimistic, helping others in need, and never revealing anything but positivity in her life. So why would such an outgoing person develop cancer? Where did the toxic emotions come into play?

A few months later, Laurel was invited to a holiday party. She overheard physicians discussing the high recurrence rate of pancreatic cancer. It had the lowest survivability of any cancer with a long-term prognosis dismal at best. Those words were seared into her subconscious. Laurel attempted to put those 'toxic' words out of her thoughts, but unbeknownst to her; they were already imprinted into her mind. I equate it to an emotional abscess, continuously oozing the fear of inevitable demise to her cells. In speaking to her, I could tell by the tone in her voice that her optimism had turned to uncertainty.

It was approximately six months later (on Mother's Day), that Laurel called to tell me the cancer had returned, and it was far more aggressive than the previous occurrence. She was once again given the prognosis of death, but this time she surrendered to the diagnosis, and planned for her inevitable departure. Saddened by the news, I asked her if she ever believed she was truly cancer free. Laurel told me that the conversation she overheard was life altering, shattering her new found beliefs. She began to fear the return of the cancer, and subconsciously her body began to act as such. What she didn't understand was the program of past images were held in her subconscious mind, and regarded the events as such, so her body responded accordingly even though she was perfectly healthy at the time. I was still pondering the underlying causation that became the catalyst for the occurrence and resurgence of the disease in such a positive person.

In her final weeks, Laurel and I spoke candidly about her past, and she unearthed feelings of anger, hurt, resentment, and regret that she had been suppressing for a long time. This side of Laurel had never been revealed to me. For years she had been silently seething about family issues. Afraid to rock the boat, she buried those feelings under false smiles, pretending they no longer mattered. However, subconsciously, she was storing irritation in her cells, and what appeared to be a calm demeanor was actually harboring turmoil on the inside. It was only a matter of time before her body could no longer protect itself, and the assault on her defense system became overwhelming. You see, cells are either in growth or protection mode until their resistance ceases. This is when disease can more easily develop. It was in the finality of her life that she was able to understand how the quiet cycle of anger, hurt, rage, all these years of pent-up negative emotions and self-doubt, had contributed to her illness. She died at home surrounded by family and friends.

Laurel's death was a turning point for me. I experienced first-hand the effects of toxic emotions on a healthy body, and the devastation that transpired. I began to explore the relationship between organs in the body and the emotional aspects related to them. Was there a direct correlation between our emotions and the health of our body?

Depending on the sources (and there are a myriad of opinions and views), various neurologists speculate that we receive anywhere between 12,357 to 60,000 thoughts per day. This data is based upon the neurological function of each individual. But even more staggering is the information that Princeton Anomalies Research Program or (PEARS), has been collecting on this research for over twenty three years. PEARS suggest that if we have one thought every fifteen seconds, and sleep for approximately eight hours every evening, that would amount to 240 thoughts per minute, 14,400 per hour, or 230,000 per day. Fortunately, most are not conscious thoughts, but rather subconscious ones, which do not continuously interfere with our daily activities. Nevertheless, subconscious thoughts are vital, and a number of scientists believe these thoughts are of greater importance in our daily lives than conscious ones. According to P.E.A.R.S, we are only cognizant of approximately five percent of conscious thoughts. The remainders are subconscious and continually downloading, running silently in the background of our mind.

My view is that most of us are unaware of the important role that our thoughts, feelings, and emotions play in determining the decisions we choose everyday, particularly the ones that arise from the subconscious. And even more importantly, how negative or toxic emotions can wreak havoc not only on our mind, but our body and spirit as well, creating illness, and disease.

There are numerous variations of toxic emotions and here are a few:

1. Hurt: Victimization, offended
2. Sadness: Self-Pity, sorrow, and depression
3. Hopelessness: Lonely, despair
4. Shame: Embarrassment, disgrace
5. Fear: Anxiety, panic, dread
6. Anger: Resentment
7. Hate: Vengeful
8. Jealousy: Envy, possessiveness
9. Greed: Self-indulgence
10. Guilt: Self-blame, self-reproach

Do you recognize yourself in any of these variations? We all have experienced them at certain times in our life, but the key is learning to manage our reaction to them and not to stay in that mode.

All of these emotions, to any degree, have the potential to cause a disruption in your body, because as they expand, they begin to create a life of their own, shifting actual reality into one of detachment and solitude. By ignoring them, these emotions are forced deeper into the cells of our body, silently waiting to erupt when the environment because too toxic or overwhelmed. Emotions need to be acknowledged, addressed and released.

Most everyone has heard of the placebo effect, that is when a patient is given a sugar pill assuming it is a pharmaceutical drug, thus the patient reacts according to the 'belief' that the pill has the ability to heal, and they do. There have been numerous studies on the placebo effect, including one in 2002 by Dr. Irving Kirsch, a psychology professor at the University of Connecticut. Dr. Kirsch found that approximately eighty percent of the effects of anti-depressants measured in the lab were attributed to the placebo effect.

Conversely, negative beliefs have the ability to trigger a *Nocebo* (Latin translation: *I will harm*) effect. The *nocebo* effect is a term to describe an ill-effect caused by a suggestion or belief that something is harmful. In 2003, the Discovery Channel aired a program called 'Placebo, Mind over Medicine.' One segment featured Dr. Clifton Meador, a physician who had been haunted by the nocebo effect for twenty-nine years. He treated a patient, Sam Londe in 1974 for cancer of the esophagus, informing him that his prognosis was grim, and the disease has a very high mortality rate. A few weeks later, Mr. Londe died; however the autopsy revealed that his esophagus was fine. He had a few spots on his liver, and one on his lung, but certainly not enough to cause his demise. Dr. Meador said that the patient died *with* cancer but not *from* cancer and if he had not given that terminal prognosis, would Sam Londe still be alive? Was the implication of inevitable death the basis for his demise, since clearly the cancer was not the causation? You see, our biology adapts to our beliefs and that is the source to understanding the powerful influence of our mind and creation. We can choose to live in fear, or love. One allows our cells to be more susceptible to disease, the other to well-being. The proverbial glass half full or half empty theory is not just an aphorism; it is the recipe to a healthy, productive life. One acronym for FEAR is: False Expectations Appearing Real. Choose to live in love rather than fear significantly transforms those beliefs. I like to equate the word emotion as: E = energy in motion.

Louise Hay, a skilled motivator, founder of Hay House Publishing and author of 'You Can Heal Your Life', believes that each organ holds cellular emotions. The pancreas for example was related to "*Not enjoying the sweetness of life*," as well as *"anger associated with sadness."* Both of those explanations described Laurel's emotional state for most of her adult life.

Dr. Candice Pert, a former Chief of Brain Biochemistry at the NIH (National Institute of Health) for thirteen years, feels that there is a definite connection between emotions and our health. Dr. Pert stated that emotions are not fully expressed until they reach consciousness. Until then, they are stored in the body and there is overwhelming evidence that unexpressed emotions cause illness.

In working with clients in my practice, I have learned that is that there is never a "one size fits all" protocol for everyone. I show them how to reframe their thoughts in order to change their perception. This process allows each client not only to understand the core of their perceptions, how they developed them, but more significantly, how to transform those beliefs.

Here are four important starting points that I would like to share with you:

Number One: Recognize that you are NOT a victim and powerless to your circumstances. If you are unhappy with the circumstances in your life, change your course! Only YOU can create your life. When you are able to make that internal shift, you then begin to rewrite the story of your life. Do not allow others to decide your future for you. It's your life!

Number Two: Everything that enters our life, good or bad, is only because of our perception of the situation. What this means is whatever we experience in life is only based on what we perceive as reality. If you change your perception, you change the way you see the world. Here is an example of what I mean:
Not long ago, I saw a beautiful sunset and was in awe of its beau-

ty. My neighbor saw the exact same sunset as toxic, caused by the refraction of the light on the pollution which created the amazing colors. Both were correct, with very different perceptions, and our body responded accordingly... one in fear, the other in love.

Number Three: Write it down. Whether you like to journal, or just take notes on a pad, when you physically write your issues down, you begin the process of releasing the emotions from your body. This means physically hand writing, not typing on a computer.

Have you ever written something when you are angry? Look at the way you wrote the words. The emotion is on the paper, not so when type on a keyboard. Anger is not a place to live, but rather a place to pass through. Writing allows you to do just that.

Number Four: You must BELIEVE that you are deserving, and in doing so, the power of beliefs within you will begin to rearrange your life. Do not allow the beliefs of others to control your reality. You see, reality is nothing more than the imagination claiming its beliefs to be factual. Trust your inner wisdom, for it has always been there.

Mahatma Gandhi wrote:
Your beliefs become your thoughts-
Your thoughts become your words-
Your words become your actions-
Your actions become your habits-
Your habits become your value-
Your value becomes your destiny…

What beliefs are you selecting, that will ultimately determine the outcome of your life?

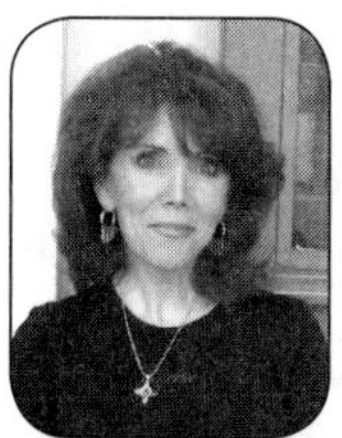

About Linda

Linda M. McCarthy, Ph.D has studied the "Mind-Body" connection for over 20 years, with a particular interest in the field of Metaphysics and Psychology. Her pursuit began while observing the significant changes in the general health of individuals as it related to their thoughts, beliefs, and emotions. Personally witnessing the physical illnesses that friends and family were experiencing, Linda began to focus her attention on the biology of beliefs, and the critical role of perception in all aspects of our life.

As a Metaphysician with a doctorate in Metaphysical Counseling and a Board Certified Life Strategist with the Spencer Institute and the American Association of Drugless Practitioners, she is currently continuing her education at Stanford University, studying Human Behavioral Biology. Linda has a passion for pursuing the deep personal connection between emotions and how they affect the well-being of an individual through energetic pathways in the body.

Her research at the University of Arizona, and University of Sedona include the exploration of biology, metaphysics and counseling, with an emphasis on the mind-body connection.

Linda McCarthy can be found in So Scottsdale Magazine, and has written numerous articles for *Evolution Ezine Magazine*. She has been a guest on the popular radio show Networking AZ. KNFX, with Carol Blonder, and is an active member of the Arizona Holistic Chamber of Commerce, The Institute of Noetic Sciences, and has a busy practice based in Scottsdale AZ.

To learn more about Linda M. McCarthy, Ph.D, and how you can receive your free phone consultation, please visit : www.newdirectioncoaching.com or call: (480) 477-8020.

CHAPTER 3

Bad Habits Be Gone

By Mallory Cargile

When I was a new trainer with a pocketful of dreams and a head full of exercises, I thought that all of my clients at Tuscaloosa Adventure Boot Camp, were going to get healthy and reach their goals. Through my workouts, nutrition seminars, and daily motivation, I was giving them all the tools they needed. How could they not? But as the saying goes, you can lead the horse to water, but you can't make him stop eating cheese fries. I can offer my clients major calorie-killer workouts, hundreds of recipes, tips on losing weight, and advice on making small changes that lead to big results. What I realized, though, was that no matter how much information I give them, if they aren't ready and willing to put in the work to change habits, all I can do is hold out hope for them. Keep encouraging them, give them advice, and hold out hope that they will get out of their comfort zone in order to make a really big change in their lives. When they finally get to that point, and when I can literally see it happening, it reminds me how much I love my job. I may have provided guidance but they made the decision to finally do something. They made the decision to change habits.

We all know we are supposed to have healthy habits. There are constant reminders of the consequences of poor health, from doctors on television to the alarming number of sweatpants being worn at the mall food court. So if we know we need to make changes, why don't we? Why are we still eating food that isn't really food, drinking soda, smoking, and skipping our exercise? One word…HABIT.

The definition of a habit is *"an acquired behavior pattern regularly followed until it has become almost involuntary." The key word here is "involuntary."* Whether it is a good or a bad habit, it is just a part of our routine. Routines are comfortable. They are familiar. In the chaos of our daily lives, they give us a sense of peace and contentment. But what if your current routine was replaced by a healthier one? Even though it's new and different at first, wouldn't it be worth it to try and make that our new normal?

Changing a habit is not easy. If it were, drug addicts would never relapse, no one would be overweight, and we would all wake up early enough to get in a good workout before heading to work. We would never eat junk food, and we would drink a lot of water. Studies have shown that simple habits can take an average of two months to develop and more involved habits may take even longer. Changing a habit is far from easy. But the easiest route is seldom the most effective route. It's time to take a detour.

We have become addicted to instant gratification. If I am hiking through the woods and suddenly want to listen to *Ice Ice Baby*, my phone has got my back. While this is beneficial in many facets of our life, this addiction tends to make us want everything else to happen fast, too. Even things that aren't supposed to be quick, like weight loss. Everyone wants that quick fix. I get questions from potential clients all the time like, "Can I lose 30 pounds in your 4-week boot camp?" My response is, "Not if you are doing it the right way, you won't. It's not healthy to lose that amount in 4 weeks. There is no way you gained that 30 pounds in four weeks. But if you are consistent with your workouts, and you have healthy habits outside of camp, the weight will come off the *right* way." Too many people in our culture just aren't satisfied with that. They forget how long it took them to gain that weight in the first place and then expect it to just fall right off. Why else would all of the popular, conventional diets out there be multi-million dollar businesses? They promise to help you drop the weight in record time. It usually works, too. If you are drastically cutting calories or cutting out food groups, of course you will lose the weight. It may surprise you to hear, however, that these businesses as a whole have a 90% fail rate with maintaining the weight loss.

Unfortunately, many people just see it as a brief phase they have to suffer through before they can start living their life again. The focus is on how quick they can lose it, not how they will maintain it. The reason there is so much failure is because most people don't learn anything. They don't....change habits. When they run out of the food shipped to their door or they stop taking those pills, they are back at square one and with a much thinner wallet.

Think of a habit in your life you want to change. Poor eating, not exercising, not getting enough sleep, smoking, drinking, whatever it is, I know you have thought about breaking that habit. If not, you wouldn't be reading this. Maybe you have more than one that you would like to change. But it's not enough to want to change the habit. Unlike gifts, it isn't the thought that counts. You have to be willing to put the work in to change it. You have to get out of that comfy routine and get over the threshold. The threshold is the time it takes to form the habit until it becomes your NEW comfy routine. Pretty soon, these new habits will be the things you miss when you have an off day and they don't happen. When you just can't fit in exercise one day, something really feels missing. THAT is when you know the habit is formed. You can then sleep better at night knowing that you are living well... and because you are exhausted from getting up at 5 a.m. to run four miles.

Whatever bad habits you are trying to break, here are ten tips on how to kick 'em to the curb and say hello to a healthier you.

1) **Never leave a black hole where your bad habit used to reside.** You always want to have a healthy habit locked and loaded to replace it. If you want to stop eating junk out of the vending machine, make sure to bring a healthy snack and have it about the same time each day. Maybe even go outside to eat it on a nice day. If having two glasses of wine is your usual nighttime ritual and you want to stop, be sure to start a new nighttime ritual that you enjoy. Some decaf herbal tea may not sound as fun but you would be surprised. It's very soothing, and you will certainly feel better the next day.

2) **Be honest with yourself about your weaknesses.** Everyone has them. I know that my weakness is that if it's in the house, I will eat it. If I have leftover cookies or cake after a party, I have to throw it away immediately or I wind up a sobbing mess, lying on the floor wracked with stomach pains and guilt from the cake in my belly and the frosting in my hair. I have even gone so far as to spray cleaner on it. Yep, whatever works. Do you eat out too much? Do you spend a lot of time and money in the fast food drive thru? Are you often groggy because you can't stop staying up too late watching mindless television? Has it been a while since you did any physical activity? Whatever it is, be honest with yourself. If not, you are in denial, and denial is not your friend.

3) **Work on one habit at a time.** It can be overwhelming if you try to change too much at one time. While it's great that you recognize all of the changes you need to make, make sure you master one before you take on another.

4) **Be aware of your environment.** A habit, whether good or bad, is usually associated with certain places, people, or activities. If you are trying to stop smoking, steer clear of your smoker friends for a while. If you want to lose weight and have friends who love to go out for beer, burgers and fries, they are probably not who you need to be having dinner with right now. You can't set yourself up for failure and expect to succeed.

5) **Be realistic.** If you are trying to create a habit of exercising 5 days per week, that's phenomenal. The benefits of that are endless. Just be sure to be realistic about the outcome. If you want the result to be that you lose 30 pounds in a month, you are setting yourself up for failure and disappointment. A healthier way to approach it would be, "Every time I lose another 5 pounds, I am going to reward myself with a new dress." For the men out there, how about a round of golf at your favorite course? Rewarding yourself for reaching specific milestones (that you need to have written down, by the way), is a great way to stick to your plan.

6) **Having a good support system is key.** Who better to have your back than your immediate family? They love you and are also often with you. Make them aware of what you are trying to do and also any help you need from them. I bet you also know someone else, a co-worker or a friend, who wants to make some healthy changes, too. Take a yoga class together, go on walks during your lunch hour, and keep each other in check. When you feel that someone is in it with you, it makes a world of difference.

7) **This one applies to those wanting to change their diet.** First, STOP using the word "diet". Unfortunately, the word has taken on a whole new meaning over the years. Before it got a bad rap, your "diet" was just how and what you eat. Now, it's one of those dreaded four-letter-words. Diets have an end point. You are going to do this or that diet for 30 days. Well....then what? We can't help that the connotation of the word has changed. Since it has, let's use a different paradigm. Immediately replace the word "diet" with the word "lifestyle." Your lifestyle doesn't have an end point. This is just how you eat now. Second, don't be so strict with your new lifestyle that you aren't happy. If you eat cottage cheese and celery sticks all day, you are not going to be happy. Chances are you won't stick to it. There is so much healthy food out there that tastes amazing and that makes you feel satisfied. Find what works

for you and stick to it! Remember, diets don't work. Good habits do.

8) **Once you have begun your new healthy habit, REPEAT… REPEAT… REPEAT!** And then repeat again. The more you repeat your healthy habit, the sooner it will become part of you. The sooner it becomes a part of you, the easier it will be to stay on track when you have a bad day or a bad week. One of my favorite clients told me that after three years of working with me, she is finally to a point where she isn't scared to go on vacation or miss a week of workouts when she absolutely has to do so. It is a part of her now. She misses it when she is gone, and she returns ready to rock. If you can get to that point, you are golden.

9) **Be selfish. Yep, that's right.** It's not only okay to be selfish sometimes, it's necessary for your physical and mental well being. Women especially tend to take on the role of taking care of everyone and everything else, leaving no room to take care of themselves. I once had a woman call me who was dying to sign up for one of my boot camp sessions. She has eight kids, is stressed to the max, and never takes time for herself. She registered on my website, and I was expecting to see her bright and early Monday morning. She was a no-show and later told me that she felt too selfish being away from the house to exercise for an hour. My classes are at 5:30 am so her children would be asleep during her workouts. She said although they would never know she was gone, she felt too guilty. This was so disappointing because I cannot imagine how stressful it is to have eight children, and I know she would have really benefited from the mental boost that came from the exercise. Everyone should make it a habit to have a little "me-time" every day, even if just for 10 minutes. Just make sure it's a healthy "me-time." Sneaking off for a cigarette or a triple-whip mocha frappucino is not the way to go. What people don't realize is that taking time for yourself each day, whether that is for exercise, reading a book, or just sitting

in a quiet room and drinking tea, will do wonders for you. I know for me, it makes me a better wife, mother, and friend.

10) **Stop saying you don't have time:** time to prepare healthy meals, time to be active, time to put in the work to stop smoking or drinking, time to get enough sleep. Here's the truth. No one HAS time. We are all busy. People who make their health and wellness a priority? They MAKE the time. You make time for your favorite television shows. You make the time to go out to dinner with family and friends. So make the time to work on you.

Remind yourself that you only get one life. There are no do-overs. Is it high enough on your priority list to focus on your health and your longevity? I hope the answer is yes, because you deserve it, and you are worth it.

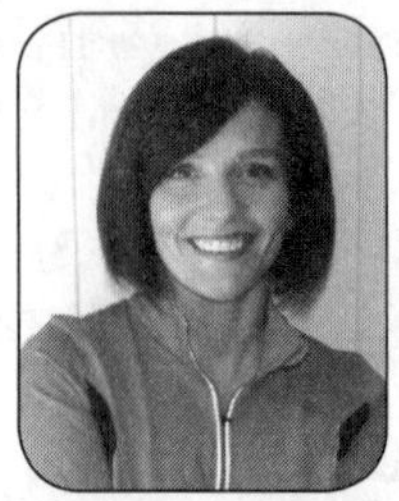

About Mallory

Mallory Cargile is the owner of Tuscaloosa Adventure Boot Camp, LLC, in Tuscaloosa, Alabama. She is a NESTA certified Personal Fitness Trainer, Boot Camp Instructor, Fitness Nutrition Coach, and Food Psychology Coach. Mallory has been featured on ABC, CBS, NBC, and FOX affiliates, as well as local newspapers and magazines, as a leading expert in health and fitness. She is often sought out by the media to give her opinion on topics ranging from exercise to healthy eating and improving vitality and longevity.

Mallory has many years of experience not only with hands-on teaching but also writing about health topics. With a degree in journalism, Mallory is dedicated to reaching out to others through various publications as well as her health and wellness blog at www.healthtotheknow.com. Mallory and her husband, Craig, founded this blog to promote wellness with an entertaining twist.

Before beginning her full-time fitness career, Mallory was a pharmaceutical representative who taught fitness classes on the side. She fell in love with teaching fitness, but soon felt conflicted that she was promoting health and wellness to her class participants but was then promoting products that provided the band-aid, not the solution. She quit her job and decided she wanted to put 100% of her focus into helping others prevent themselves from ever needing that blood pressure medication or that diabetes insulin. She wanted to be a part of the solution and often reminds her clients that exercising and eating healthy is not just for your waistline. It's about longevity and quality of life.

Mallory is extremely passionate about helping others realize that making small changes in their lives lead to big results. She has a strong track record of helping people increase confidence, relieve stress, fit into those jeans in the back of the closet, and realize that it's necessary to make it a priority to focus on health every day.

She lives in Centreville, Alabama, with her husband, Craig, and their sons, George and Vann.

If you are interested in online personal training, how to shop healthy in the

grocery store, safe products Mallory recommends, or want to join her local Adventure Boot Camp, please visit: www.tuscaloosabootcamp.com or call 205-391-8588.
www.tuscaloosabootcamp.com
www.healthtotheknow.com
www.mallorycargile.com

CHAPTER 4

Mastering Your Body

By Briar Munro

My name is Briar Munro and I own Fly Girl Fitness in Toronto, Canada. I first decided to get into the fitness/health industry when I was twelve years old. It was at that age that I was diagnosed with Legg-Calve-Perthes Disease. This is a degeneration of the bones of my hip. I spent many hours at Sick Kids Hospital and had my first surgery just months after my diagnosis.

I was told that because I was diagnosed so late that until my surgery I shouldn't be walking and that I should be in a wheel chair. As a twelve year old dancer and martial artist this was not good news! As you can imagine it was a very trying time for myself and my family.

When I was doing my physiotherapy after my surgery I decided that the health care field was where I wanted to be. I wanted to help others with their health related problems to live healthier, happier lives.

One thing I have come to learn through my studies and my own life is that being healthy doesn't just mean exercising and eating "healthy" foods. It means living a healthy lifestyle. I have spent the past few years transitioning myself and helping my clients go through the transition of living more holistically.

Living holistically means realizing that all parts of our life need to be taken into consideration. Our needs psychologically, physically, socially, and mentally are acknowledged and treated as equal parts. Also, there is an understanding that each of those parts affects all the others. For example, if we are depressed or have a chronic injury, all our systems are affected and we could see other problems arise.

There are five main topics that need to be discussed to master your body. Let's go through them each now.

1. MOTIVATION AND GOALS

This may seem like an odd thing to be looking at when talking about our health. However, if we don't have a clear vision for where we want to go in our lives then what's the point in being healthy? We need to have a dream, a vision for our future in order to motivate us to move forward, to get up each day.

So what is your dream? What makes you happy? What do you want to achieve while you are on this earth? If you were to die tomorrow what would you like to leave behind? How would you like your friends and family to describe you?

Still not sure what your dream is? That's okay. Let's look at your core values. What do you stand for? What's important to you? What do you believe in? Having a dream gives us direction and motivates us to continue our journey.

2. UNDERSTANDING FOOD AND DIGESTION

Often when we are trying to get healthy, we think we have to eat only fruits and vegetables. However, what we eat isn't nearly as important as the quality of our food.

I believe that the way our lives have changed over the years has really impacted the way we eat. For instance, we are expected to work 9-14 hours per day as opposed to the old average of 8 hours. It is expected that we will be available to be contacted 24 hours per day with all of our new technology, and if we don't respond we are being rude or bad business people. Our children are taking 3-5 different after-school activities so that they are considered more "well-rounded." We are so busy that we no longer have time to make home-cooked meals or grocery shop. In fact, our stores had to change to being open 24 hours per day because we couldn't figure out how to get there during regular business hours.

We are in a state of chaos and our bodies are paying the toll. We are relying on caffeine, fast food, pre-cooked, and ready-made meals to sustain us, along with foods that should not be available to us at certain times of the year.

This is my favorite food saying…

If your grandparents didn't eat it, then neither should you!

Our grandparents were brought up on home cooked meals that were prepared the same day and often from ingredients that were bought that day (sometimes even directly from the farmers). It was part of their daily routine. There were no processed foods that lasted on our shelves for months at a time. There were no fast-food restaurants to run into. Instead, there was a set time for a family dinner each night that everyone made it home for. Kids started their day with real food, rather than sugary, processed cereals or pop tarts. If you keep this thought in the forefront of your mind, then you will really see a change to what you are eating and therefore to a lot of other parts of your health and wellbeing.

Next lets talk about organic foods. The difference between organic foods and commercially raised or produced foods are huge! Nutrients are what give our foods their taste. Organic foods won't look as good but they will taste much better and have 'way more' nutrients.

One of the things commercial farmers do is they put so much salt on the ground that the plants have to suck up huge amounts of water to neutralize the salt and survive. This makes for bigger, lovely looking produce, but in reality you get big empty corncobs and big empty carrots.

In fact to get the same nutrition from one head of lettuce as you did 50 years ago, you'd have to eat 20 heads of lettuce from the commercial farms.

Our health really comes down to the health of the soil. Commercially-raised foods are sick due to the chemicals that they are raised with. If the food cells are sick, we will be sick as well. Whatever the farmer does to the soil affects the end result of everyone who eats those crops (animals included!).

If our food is no longer natural and is modified, how do you think your systems will deal with it? Our body is not designed to digest and absorb commercially-made chemicals. The degree to which our digestive system is deficient equals the degree to which our energy system is deficient.

What is the difference between organic and certified organic? Organic means that there were no sprays, pesticides or chemicals of any kind used to grow those foods. Certified organic also means that there are proper crop rotations done and that the company or farm is being monitored to ensure that it is organic.

Proper crop rotation means that the farmer will plant dissimilar crops in the same field each year so that the soil can replenish the nutrients that were depleted due to the type of crop that was grown the year previously. The soil holds so many nutrients, vitamins and minerals that are essential not only to the plant but to us as well.

Just 60 to 100 years ago, people weren't overweight because their food wasn't sick and they were moving a lot more. Doing laundry by hand was exercise. Cooking from scratch was more taxing and therefore meant more movement, there were fewer cars and therefore people walked more.

The food was much less processed and fewer chemicals were used to grow our foods. Cooking and processing extract nutrients from our foods. Food processing started around the time of WWI in order to make food last longer – so it could be shipped to our troops and so that those of us not at war would have food that we could store for longer periods at home.

Vitamins and supplements were introduced around this time (as our food was so deficient), and in fact the government made it mandatory for companies to fortify our food (like milk and bread), so that we were getting enough nutrients from our processed foods. It is fortified because it is dead. We are eating dead food, which is going to kill us!

3. STRESS AND SLEEP

Stress and sleep play a huge role in our overall health. If you are stressed and/or not getting enough sleep (or recovery time) your body will react in many ways. Shutting down or getting the flu are the common ones, but did you know that spraining your ankle, constipation, night sweats, inflammatory conditions, depression, and incontinence could also be symptoms?

You have to cycle stress and recovery, and not just in terms of exercise. Let me give you an example. If you're drinking ten cups of coffee a day, that's the equivalent of working out ten times a day, and you wouldn't do that. If you cut half of that out and every second cup of coffee is replaced with water, now you're cycling stress and recovery.

Finding activities that you love to do count as recovery: Photography, writing, reading, light walking, scrapbooking are all great examples – anything that doesn't raise your heart rate.

Setting an evening routine can really help when it comes to the quality of your sleep. Spend an hour before bed calming down, with low lights, hot water with lemon, a relaxing book and stretches. This tells your body it's time to prepare for sleep. Getting to bed by 10 pm and waking at 6 am will have your body functioning with the circadian rhythms of the earth and you will feel more rested.

Also, making sure your room is pitch black (you shouldn't be able to see your hand in front of your face), and removing all electronics from your room will help your sensory receptors to relax. Also remember to never do strenuous exercise or drink alcohol late at night, and avoid caffeine after 3 pm as these are all stimulants.

4. MOVEMENT

Movement is very important for our everyday bodily functions. We need movement to pump our blood through our body, keep our heart and lungs healthy, keep our digestive system working properly and keep our mind sharp. However, if we overdo our exercise, we can have serious repercussions.

Have you ever gone to a fitness class or worked with a trainer whose main concern is to work you so hard that you can't move the next day? What would happen if their main goal was to give you a good workout, in a safe environment where your form and technique were first priority? Wouldn't that be refreshing?

In fact, exercising adds more stress to our bodies and remember what stress can do to us? So we have to be really careful about how hard we are working out on any given day. Some days, if our psychological or spiritual aspects are too overwhelmed, it might not be a good idea to exercise at all. Stretching, foam rolling, doing meditation or tai chi-type movements might be the way to go. Exercising hard and getting your heart rate up is important too. Don't eliminate your regular exercise, just make sure you have a balance of recovery exercise as well.

The trick here is in listening to your body and deciding what it needs that day. Pushing past or working through our issues can lead to injuries. Take a moment before your next full workout and double check what your body is asking for.

5. ENVIRONMENT

Our environment (especially living in a large city) can really take a toll on our overall health and wellbeing. The toxins in the air we breathe, in our foods, from our cars, furniture and our water, are affecting us everyday.

Our detoxification system has to work extremely hard to neutralize the toxic properties of all these substances. The organs of our detoxification system include our lungs, large intestines, skin, liver and kidneys.

When the liver and kidneys are overburdened, toxins back up into the body. Spending time on breathing, exercising, skin brushing, and drinking lots of clean water from glass containers can help to balance some of the toxins we take in everyday. Also, do a tour of your house and office and see what things can be cleaned, gotten rid of or replaced with a healthier, more natural or organic version. Look at furniture, carpets, cookware, containers, cleaning products, toiletries, clothing, foods, ventilation systems, and office supplies. Next increase your levels of anti-oxidant rich foods, organic foods and clean sources of water. Decrease your exposure to chemicals, and avoid alcohol.

That may seem like a lot of information. Lets do a quick recap of what steps you should take to start on your health journey.

1. Determine your dream. Your motivation for getting up each day. What you want to achieve.

2. Start being aware of the quality of your foods. Choose natural, organic foods and avoid anything processed or foods sprayed with chemicals. Remember, if it lasts on your shelf longer than a week or two, it probably isn't good for you. Also, if your grandparents didn't eat it, neither should you!

3. Cycle your stress and sleep so that you are better balanced. Clear your bedroom and prepare an hour or so

before bed for optimal sleep. Find activities that you love that will help you to relax

4. Listen to your body. If you are already overstressed, exercising might not be the best idea. Spend your time on deep breathing, stretching, foam rolling, tai chi or swimming.

5. Do an environment overhaul and see what you can clear or replace, so that your detoxification system isn't on overload.

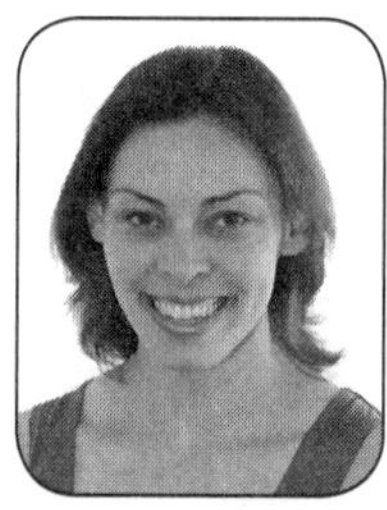

About Briar

Briar Munro is a fitness professional from Toronto, Canada. With a background in dance and martial arts, Briar has taken her love for athletics and personal health and turned it into a unique approach to personal training and health education.

Briar holds a diploma from George Brown College from their 3 year Fitness and Lifestyle Management program. She is certified as a Personal Trainer from Can Fit Pro, certified as a Physiotherapy Assistant from Robotech Institute Inc, is a certified Stott Pilates instructor and dance teacher, as well as holds a Level 2 Holistic Lifestyle Coach from the C.H.E.K. Institute. Her company, Fly Girl Fitness, combines traditional personal training methodology and Pilates technique with holistic lifestyle coaching to address the health of the whole person, body and mind, and to achieve fitness, health and life goals. For Briar, it is not just about reaching a desired weight or adding more muscles, but about the ability to live the healthiest life possible, which will ultimately result in weight loss, muscle gain, longevity and happiness.

You can reach Briar at 416-671-4399, briar@flygirlfitness.com or learn more about her programs and philosophy on her website: www.flygirlfitness.com

CHAPTER 5

The Art of Breathing

Reduce stress and tension in less than 10 minutes per day

By Lisa Fox Bail, CK

What would you think if I told you that you could improve your life just by performing a handful of simple breathing exercises for a few minutes each day? Wouldn't it be great if it were that simple? Well it is! We take an average of 20,000 breaths per day, so imagine the impact that changing your breathing can have.

Let me start off by telling you my story. As an adolescent I was a competitive gymnast. I spent many long hours in the gym focusing on my body – perfecting my form and constantly striving to improve my strength and flexibility. I was no stranger to the pain and hard work it took to push my body to do what I wanted it to do. Then one day when I was 16, I woke up in the middle of the night in extreme pain. I had scoliosis (a curve in my spine), which had become unstable causing several herniated discs as a result. After several tests, my doctor recommended that I have surgery as soon as possible to correct the curve and minimize any long term nerve damage. During the surgery they cut my back open and attached two metal rods to my spine. This straightened me out but left more than half of my spine immobile.

Almost overnight I went from super flexible to barely able to put on my own shoes. I knew that the recovery from such major surgery would be difficult, but I wasn't worried since I was used to pushing my body and working through pain. And, as expected, the pain from surgery eased after several weeks but another pain crept in above and below where the surgery had been. Instead of getting stronger, I began feeling weaker and my posture was getting worse. By just a few months after my surgery I was terribly hunched over and completely unable to straighten up. I had also developed chronic pain and was pretty frustrated and miserable. I returned to my surgeon and he informed me that I had arthritis, which was to be expected after the type of surgery that I had. Basically, the areas of my spine above and below where the rods were had to take so much strain due to such a large part of my back being immobile that they were wearing out. I was devastated to get such news before I had even turned twenty. My surgeon told me that there was nothing that I could do except take medication for the pain and once it got bad enough then I could have more surgery. Since surgery was what caused the chronic pain that I was currently experiencing I did not think that more surgery was the right solution.

Right then I made a decision: I was going to figure out how to make my body feel better. I knew that I needed to get my strength and flexibility back and I figured yoga could help so I bought a book about yoga and started working through some of the exercises. There really wasn't much I could do at first and most things that I tried caused me a lot of pain so I focused instead on the breathing exercises. That is when everything started to turn around. As I began to breathe better, I found that my body began to soften and become more pliable. As I began to breathe better, I found that I could do some of the poses gently without pain. As I began to breathe better, I found that I was able to remain in one position for longer periods. As I began to breathe better, I started to be more optimistic, my mood improved, and I had more energy. As I began to breathe better, I started to get my life back. Today I am an active mother and fitness professional. I have very few limitations and I am happy to say that I can now bend over and touch my toes.

Not everyone has experienced such a major issue with their body, but all of the clients that I have worked with have experienced noticeable benefits from doing a few simple exercises to improve their breathing. Since breathing occurs continually without conscious thought, it is something that most people rarely pay any attention to. As a result of stress, previous injury or illness, an inactive lifestyle, or a number of other factors, most people have developed habits or compensations over time, which impairs their ability to breathe efficiently and effectively. Second only to our heart beating, breathing is the most important function in our body. We can go weeks without eating, days without drinking, but we can only survive for a few minutes without breathing.

Here are the basics of breathing: when you breathe in, air enters the lungs and when you breathe out, air leaves the lungs. I'm guessing you already knew that part but did you ever wonder how that happens? It is actually caused by the muscles surrounding the lungs, which change the pressure inside of the lungs causing air to either enter or leave the lungs. Most of this comes from the diaphragm which contracts downward when you breathe in, pulling the bottom of the lungs with it causing negative pressure in the lungs and drawing in air from outside your body to balance the pressure. The diaphragm is attached to the lower ribs and low back and separates the torso into upper and lower halves with the heart and lungs above and the abdominal organs below. Diaphragmatic breathing massages the abdominal organs and causes a relaxation response in the body, slowing the heart rate and relieving tension.

With optimal breathing, the diaphragm contracts downwards as you breathe in, pulling on the lower ribs and drawing them downward, causing the belly to expand. When you breathe out, the diaphragm relaxes and the belly softens as the ribs returns to their resting position. However, many people have altered breathing patterns so that when they breathe in, the belly and/ or ribs don't move and instead the shoulders rise up to allow the lungs to expand. This type of breathing creates tension in the neck and shoulder muscles and causes the release of stress hormones making you feel anxious and uneasy.

So now that you know this, let's check how you're breathing. Try this simple self assessment: place one hand on your abdomen over your belly button and place your other hand on your chest. Take a few breaths in and out. What do you feel? You should feel the hand on your abdomen rising and falling with your breath and very little movement under the hand on your chest. Now take breath that is a little bigger than normal. What do you feel this time? You should still feel the hand on your abdomen rising as the belly expands outwards then as you fill your lungs more completely the ribs will expand out to the sides and the chest will rise slightly, however, the shoulders should not lift and the neck and jaw should remain relaxed. If this is not what you felt, then I recommend that you spend 10 minutes each day practicing the breathing exercises in this chapter and you will be amazed at how the tension begins to drain from your body and you are able to move through your days with more energy and less pain.

Caution: Please respect your body and do not do anything that causes any amount of pain or discomfort. These exercises are intended to be very gentle and safe, however, I cannot ensure that they are appropriate for everybody. In all cases the breath should be smooth, easy, and continuous.

DIAPHRAGMATIC BREATHING – 2 MINUTES

This exercise is basically what is described in the first part of the self-assessment above. Even if you passed this test with flying colors it is still beneficial to spend a few minutes each day focusing on breathing this way because our breathing can get thrown out of whack occasionally and become irregular (such as when we get stressed or are sick). You will need to master this exercise before moving on to the others.

How to do it: This exercise can be performed in any position but usually people are most comfortable lying on their back. Place one hand on the abdomen and the other on your chest. As you breathe in allow the belly to expand, feeling the hand rise while keeping your chest relaxed and minimizing any movement beneath that hand. Focus on the sensations of the breath coming down into the bottom of the lungs causing the belly to expand when you breathe in. As you breathe out, just relax and allow the air to naturally flow back out of the body. This breathing should be very relaxed and unstrained, as you are not forcing the breath but just allowing it to come and go.

Note: if you are finding it difficult to keep the chest relaxed and allowing the belly to expand then using a 'breathing bag' will be helpful – this is a cloth bag with a couple pounds of weight to it (you can make your own by filling a sock with rice). Place the bag across your lower abdomen and gently push your belly out as you breathe in to cause the bag to rise. Although we do not normally want to force the breath, this technique will get you accustomed to expansion of the belly. After a few sessions of this, you should find that you are able to allow the belly to expand on its own without pushing.

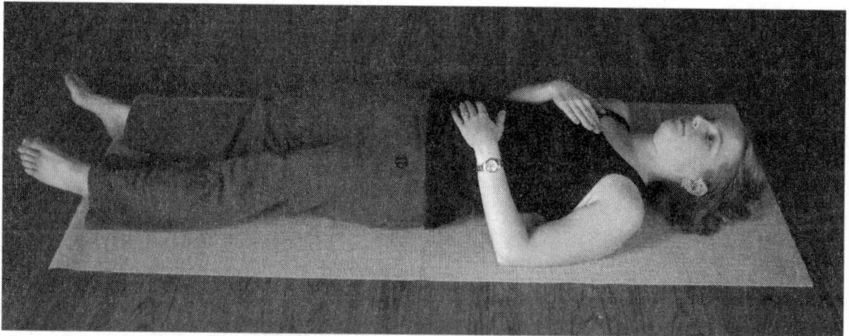

3-PART BREATH – 1 MINUTE

This exercise will teach you how to breathe when you have greater oxygen needs, such as during exercise. It also helps stretch and strengthen the breathing muscles and connective tissue around the lungs. This is the same as the second part of the self assessment exercise. It too is important to practice regularly, even once you are able to perform it flawlessly. This exercise can be performed in any position as well but you'll likely be most comfortable lying on your back.

How to do it: Continue breathing diaphragmatically with one hand on the abdomen and the other on the chest and begin to take deeper breaths. Try to fill the lungs as completely as possible, from bottom to top, while keeping the shoulders, neck and jaw relaxed. The shoulders should not rise at all during this exercise. As you breathe in, focus on the breath filling the lungs from the bottom to the top, first feeling the abdomen expand, then the lower ribs expanding out to the sides, and finally feel the chest expand and rise slightly beneath your hand. As you breathe out, just relax and allow the air to flow back out of the lungs feeling the chest fall, the ribs relax, and the belly soften.

SPINAL TWIST – 1 MINUTE PER SIDE

This exercise helps open up and stretch out the chest – people often hold a lot of tension here which will restrict expansion of the ribcage and negatively affect breathing. This exercise also helps you get accustomed to allowing the lower ribs to expand as you breathe.

How to do it: Roll on to one side with both the knees and hips bent at a 90 degree angle and place a small pillow beneath your head to keep your neck in line with your spine. Place your bottom hand on the outside of your top leg. Begin by raising the top arm up towards the ceiling while keeping the shoulders down and back (don't let them hunch up toward the ears). Once the arm is vertical with the fingers pointing toward the ceiling, begin to twist the torso and head, looking toward the hand. Keep the neck and jaw relaxed and the back of the head resting on the pillow. Do not let the knees move; they should remain stacked on top of one another. Go as far as feels comfortable and hold there for one minute before reversing the twist and rolling to the other side and repeating. While in the twist, firm the abdomen

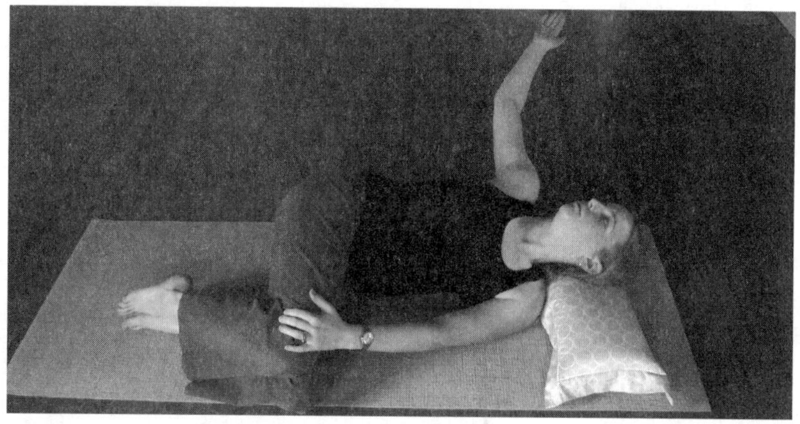

slightly and focus on directing the breath into the sides, allowing the lower ribs to gently spread apart as the ribcage expands.

CROCODILE – 1 MINUTE

When you breathe in, the lower back also expands due to the movement of the diaphragm. This exercise helps you connect with the lower back and feel the expansion there.

How to do it: Lying on your stomach, bend your arms and place your hands beneath your forehead (allowing the forehead to rest on top). Ensure that the neck is long and the back of the neck doesn't feel compressed at all. As you breathe in, focus on feeling the expansion in the lower back and noticing the lower ribs drawing back and down. This will be easier to feel if you lay on a firm surface (such as a towel or yoga mat on the floor).

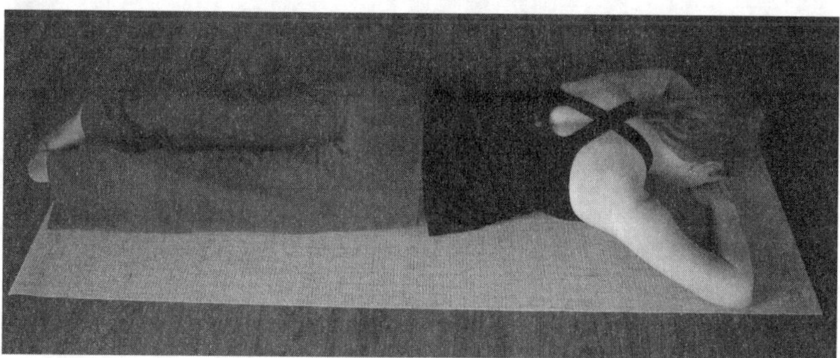

Note: If you are still having trouble feeling this then try using the breathing bag as described in the note for exercise 1. Place the bag over the back of the lower ribs (near the kidneys) and focus on directing the breath to this area. The slight weight from the breathing bag is helpful due to the feedback it provides.

ELEVATED CHILD'S POSE – 1 MINUTE

This exercise assists in stretching the muscles and connective tissue around the ribs to allow the ribs to expand more fully. It also feels lovely and is very relaxing.

How to do it: From hands and knees, bend your elbows to place your forearms on the floor, palms down. Shift your hips back slightly and rest your forehead on the floor between your elbows. Keep the shoulders down and back (not hunched up towards the ears) and the neck long to ensure that the back of the neck doesn't feel compressed. Press the inside of the elbows into the floor and maintain this pressure as you hold the position. You may feel a stretch through the arms, chest, and/or back here but it should feel relatively comfortable. Firm the abdomen slightly and direct your breath to the lower ribs and feel them expand back and to the sides, widening the ribcage as you breathe in.

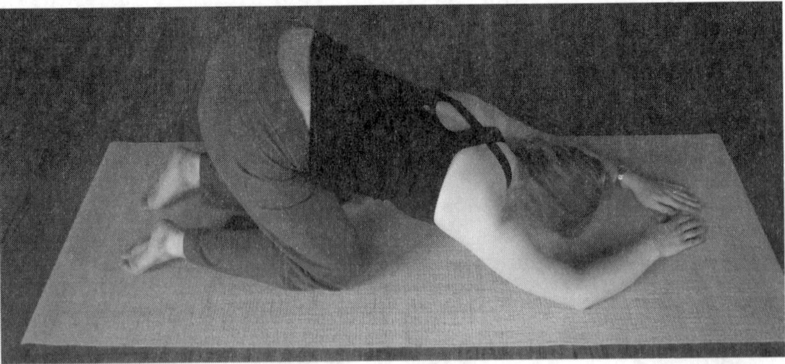

So there you are; 5 exercises that you can do in less than 10 minutes. Practice regularly (I like to do it before bed) and you will be on your way to improved breathing, less muscle tension, and lower stress. Take care and breathe well.

References:

Agur, Anne M.R. & Dalley, Arthur F. 2005. *Grant's Atlas of Anatomy, Eleventh Edition.*
Bradley, Brian. 2007. *Correct Breathing Patterns. PT on the Net.*
Hately, Susi. 2010. *Therapeutic Yoga for the Shoulders and Hips, First Edition.*
Myers, Esther. 1996. *Yoga and You: Energizing and Relaxing Yoga for New and Experienced Students.*

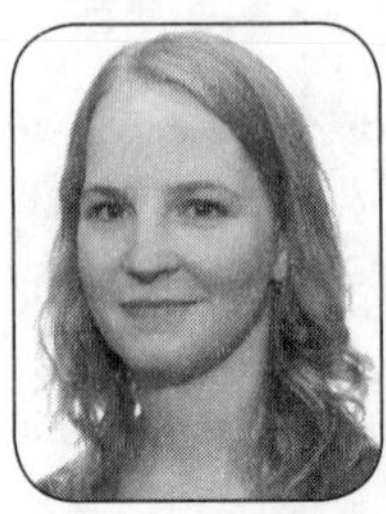

About Lisa

Lisa Fox Bail has a passion for helping people feel better and educating the public about their health. A Kinesiologist and human movement specialist, Lisa has an honors science degree from the University of Guelph. During her studies, she began helping clients as a personal trainer and then moved into a rehab setting – assisting people who had been involved in motor vehicle accidents as well as those who had experienced workplace injuries. She now combines the two disciplines and incorporates rehab activities into her training sessions. She has a thirst for knowledge and has many specialized certifications in areas such as Pilates, Pre & Post-Natal Yoga, Pre & Post-Natal Exercise, Older Adult Exercise, Nutrition & Wellness, Functional Assessment & Graduated Exercise, and Advanced Exercise Prescription.

Lisa began her own business, Health Appeal, in 2007 while looking for an innovative way to improve people's lives through health and wellness. She currently offers specialized small group classes and individual training. She especially enjoys working with pregnant women and new moms and their babies. As a mom herself she understands all of the joys and challenges that these years bring and loves to help navigate women through them. She loves nothing more than to help empower her clients to be advocates for their own health and teach them the tools they need to do so. Although Lisa lives on a farm in southwestern Ontario, Canada, she aspires to bring her message to more women via the wonders of the Internet.

Lisa regularly provides tips for moms and easily digestible health information on her blog and through social media. You can learn more about Lisa and Health Appeal by checking out her website (www.healthappeal.ca), following her on Twitter (@HealthAppeal)
or 'liking' her on Facebook (www.facebook.com/HealthAppeal).
Or just shoot her an email to Lisa@healthappeal.ca

CHAPTER 6

DANDELION DREAMS

By La-Verne Parris

"Dandelions are known to grow through concrete."
~Anonymous

Upon first meeting 40 year old Jane Doe in the winter of 2005, I was immediately struck by her fervor to change her life. Her passion for this change was palpable when she described the different root-issues she wanted to overcome. One root issue was her remaining in a 17-year off-and-on, toxic relationship with her then boyfriend, J.T. Jane had several concerns about this relationship. First, she was desperately worried that her emotional and spiritual needs were not being met. Jane was also concerned that although he professed to be "in her corner," he was obviously jealous of her, and tried to sabotage her by attacking her goals and achievements. Finally, Jane also identified an unhealthy, codependent behavioral loop that they had been involved in for almost two decades.

Another root issue that Jane wanted to change was her desire to move from teaching at the community college level to a four-year research university. Jane understood that as a professor whose research interests include cultural studies, critical race theory and existentialism, she would have access to greater resources at a four-year academic institution. She also knew that working at a four-year university would vastly improve her quality of life. In turn, she would have a more flexible work schedule that would provide her with more time to develop and formalize her own body of critical theory and complete her novel.

The last root issue that Jane acknowledged was her longing to return to the level of physical conditioning she had as a former marathoner. Jane completed three New York City Marathons in 1987, 1988 and 1989 consecutively when she was in her late 20s and turning 30. When Jane recounted the physical and emotional freedom and empowerment she felt while training for these marathons, it became obvious to me that all of Jane's self-esteem and ability to actualize was linked to her identity as an athlete. Jane later revealed that as a child she grew up extremely athletic. When she was 10 years old, Jane qualified as a Junior Lifesaver at Girl Scout Camp and grew up walking four miles back and forth to swimming lessons every summer until she was 15 years old. Once entering junior high school, Jane also joined the volleyball, field-hockey and track teams and continued playing these sports through high school. Growing up as an athlete, and as someone who always enjoyed sports, captured the happiest times in Jane's life. These moments in her life, when she felt capable of achieving anything and overcoming any and all obstacles, were always linked to Jane's identity as an athlete. It was clear to me how much Jane enjoyed feeling strong, graceful and athletic – she wanted to experience these feelings again as an adult.

Jane's last root issue was related to the satellite issue of making serious life-style changes around her relationship with food and emotional eating. Jane explained that after she completed her last marathon, her training regimen had changed, but the size of her meals had not. She was essentially eating the same amount of food, but running much fewer miles. Jane also noted that as she aged, she saw specific changes in her body's ability to digest and burn certain types of foods. As Jane approached her late twenties, she noticed that her body could no longer burn that late night bowl of cereal or digest that four a.m. tuna sandwich. She further recounted that she recognized another metabolic shift when she entered her mid-30s. Processed foods became increasingly more difficult for Jane to digest, as burgers and donuts would just sit in her stomach for hours. During our initial conversation, Jane also saw the connections among this denial of her metabolic changes, her dissatisfaction with J.T., her emotional eating, and her desire for true unconditional love.

At this point in our initial session, Jane knew three things. First, she knew that she was at a crossroads in her life around the root issues of relationships, actualizing her professional goals, and improving her health. Subsequently, having identified the root issues, Jane and I also acknowledged the existence of several satellite issues tied to these root issues. Finally, Jane also realized that by starting the life coaching process with me, she was already making serious strides in this positive direction and had begun her journey.

Since beginning our client-coach relationship, Jane has transformed herself, spiritually, personally, emotionally and professionally. Jane has completely ended her 17-year on-and-off again relationship with J.T. and is dating happily. She has also returned to her peak level of physical conditioning and maintains a healthy diet – free of processed food and excess sugar. Not only has Jane lost 40 pounds, but she also lost all the insecurities that were preventing her from taking risks in her life. Jane successfully completed and defended her dissertation; she has already had one chapter of it published in an internationally-recognized academic journal, and is expecting a second chapter publication in April 2012. Jane has also attended and presented in six academic conferences, and received invitations from colleagues to chair other panels as well. Jane is also branching out and seeking employment outside of New York for the first time in her career in academia. Lastly, and most significantly, Jane has had an excerpt from her novel published in a well-known journal of African Diaspora literature and criticism. She is currently seeking literary representation. Jane broke through her barriers, just as a dandelion has been known to grow through concrete.

10 STEPS TO SERENITY

STEP 1: Be Compassionate With Yourself and Love Yourself Unconditionally

This step lies at the heart of how we feel about ourselves and our place in the world. Make a pact with yourself to remain in a place of self-love and compassion about yourself, your feelings, your situation and your relationships. Promising that you will be loving and compassionate with yourself for all days, is the beginning of a journey that is completely free of self-judgment and self-criticism.

Very often it is so much easier for us to cheer other people on and to be a shoulder for them to cry on. We become the "ideal friend" to everyone in our lives, except ourselves. Imagine how good we could feel everyday if we said things to ourselves like: "Wow, what a great outfit!" or "Hey, great job on that presentation today!" Now is the time to discover what it could feel like to overcome challenging situations by being compassionate with yourself.

Wherever you are at this moment in your life, take a minute or two and repeat this statement:

"I love myself unconditionally. I am a good, kind and loving person. I will be patient and compassionate with myself today, and all days, as I move forward with my goals and as I move forward in my life."

Taking a minute out of each day to be positive, loving and nurturing with ourselves helps us to take control of our own thoughts and actions.

STEP 2: Keep Track of and Be Aware of Your Self-Talk

Simply put, Self-Talk is how we talk to ourselves on a daily basis. The average person has between 12,357 and 60,000 thoughts in one day. (http://www.funtrivia.com/askft/Question35395.html.) If we start out our day on a negative note without making the conscious decision to become more positive, it is likely that we will end the day on that very same negative note. However, if we start out the day acknowledging that we are feeling a little negative, but that the day could improve, then we have already lifted our feelings from a negative state to a more positive state. The key to healthy self-talk is to begin keeping track of your negative thoughts and replacing them with more loving and kind thoughts.

Negative Thoughts: I feel awful today. Why did I stay up so late last night? How am I going to make it through this day?

Positive Replacement Thoughts: I'm a little tired because I went out last night. I deserve to have a social-life. I work really hard all the time. I'll make sure that I drink lots of water and try to take get some fresh air at lunchtime.

Do you see how changing our thoughts can automatically helps us to change our mood? By changing our moods and remaining on a path of self-love and nurturing, we can begin to change specific aspects of our lives.

STEP 3: Address the Root Issues of Your Unhappiness

With compassion and positive self-talk in your arsenal, you can now begin to lovingly question yourself and examine how to become happier and more fulfilled in your life. Understand that this step is on-going, just as the other steps are; because as you continue to grow and change in your life, so will the situations and circumstances that you would like to change.

Taking the time to peacefully and patiently ask yourself: "What would I like to change in my life?" can indeed be a self-empowering moment. For it is in this moment that you can be honest with yourself about your past, present and future. You can also begin to forgive yourself for any past hurts and disappointments you have visited upon yourself and others.

During this self-examination, many root issues are revealed, as well as their connected satellite issues. Whatever your root and satellite issues are, this preliminary stage of compassionate self-inquiry is an essential part of your happiness.

STEP 4: Identify the Satellite Issues that Are Outgrowths of the Root Issue

In this step you are taking a deeper look at how your root issues have affected other areas of your life. One negative issue in our lives is usually attached to multiple satellite issues. For example, if a person's root issue is improved health and fitness and she begins her journey towards this goal by eating healthier foods, and increased exercise, she will see and feel the rewards of her hard work. She will begin to feel better about her appearance and start wearing nicer clothes, or try a new hair-style.

As she begins to feel more confident and free from insecurities, she starts attending and participating in more professional conferences. Because she has become more confident, she is increasingly taking more risks and putting herself in new situations that are benefiting her.

STEP 5: Identify the Goals You Want to Accomplish

Make a list of different short-term and long-term goals that you would like to accomplish. Creating this distinction between short-term and long-term goals allows you to understand which goals are long-term or on-going, and which goals can be realized over a shorter period of time with tangible results. Writing down your goals also allows you to see, and question, the amount of time and energy required to achieve each goal.

STEP 6: Create a Roadmap for Each Goal

Now that you have already identified your short-term and long-term goals, it is time to begin mapping out how you will reach these goals. For example, if a person's goal is to receive a promotion at his job, his roadmap should contain practical milestones that will help him get that promotion. One milestone should include a list of different academic courses and/or trade-related courses that would help him to advance professionally. Another milestone could include a list of key people in his desired field for informational interviews. The purpose of an informational interview is to speak with individuals who are currently working at your desired level and in your desired field. Hearing the experiences of others and taking note of their suggestions can be an invaluable resource for someone seeking career satisfaction.

STEP 7: Allow Yourself to Grow and Change

While you are on your journey of self-development, it is highly likely that you will release old, negative habits and negative people. As you put your energies into more positive pursuits, you will naturally have less energy for negative situations and negative people. You may notice a subtle shift in yourself and the things that you once liked to do. You may also sense yourself becoming increasingly uncomfortable around people who believe they were put on this earth solely to gossip and complain.

By giving yourself permission to react according to how you feel at this particular moment, you are acknowledging your own growth. You are also ushering in a new era in your own life that is characterized by strength and determination.

STEP 8: Acknowledge Each Milestone and Each Accomplishment

As you continue to take responsibility for your happiness, it is very important that you recognize each milestone and each accomplishment. Think back to when you were a child or young adult. Which types of celebrations did you enjoy the most? Did you have a ball at big parties? Or, did you prefer hanging out with a few close friends? Perhaps, you were the more solitary type who just loved looking up at the night sky?

Whichever celebratory scenario best fits your personality, start incorporating it every time you have completed a milestone on your roadmap or you have accomplished a goal. Get into the habit of being good to yourself by treating yourself to little things. Take a walk at lunchtime, write a poem, call an old friend, do any positive thing that makes you happy. You do deserve to be happy.

STEP 9: Be Grateful and Self Check-In

On your journey through improved well-being, it is crucial that you regularly appreciate the blessings in your life and that you monitor your feelings. Begin keeping a gratitude journal. The simple, yet powerful, act of being thankful for what you have can, over time, transform your life. By writing down the people, and things, for which you are thankful automatically changes your energy from lack to abundance.

Self check-in is a very practical and useful tool as it keeps you present in the moment. You are showing yourself kindness, consideration and compassion. Wherever you are, you can take a moment to ask yourself: "Okay, how am I feeling about this?" or "What can I do to make myself feel better right now?" Going through this quick self check-in will also help you to separate multiple issues occurring simultaneously.

STEP 10: Reevaluate Goals and Be Ready to Set New Ones

Keep an open mind about your goals. While you are becoming more positive and productive you will notice that you need to augment your goals, or put them to rest and take on new challenges.

For example, if your goal is to complete your first marathon, you may want to plan other athletic challenges you want to try after you finish the marathon.

Planning ahead helps you to maintain a positive frame of mind about your goal, and it also staves off the well-known anti-climactic feeling people experience after achieving a monumental goal.

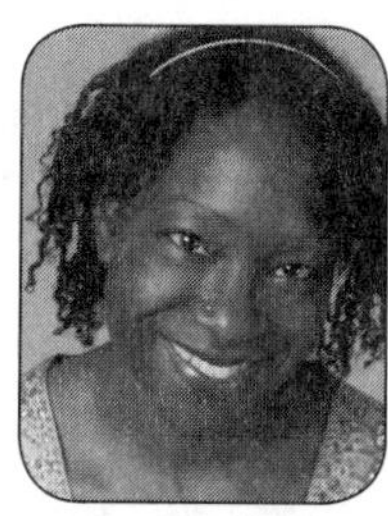

About La-Verne

La-Verne Parris, also known as the Miracle Worker, is a best selling Life coach and Educator who is regularly sought out by actors, athletes, musicians, writers and artists for her unique and uncanny ability to guide them to their next levels of self-actualization. La-Verne insists that with each client's successes, everything they have accomplished was already within them.

"I only shine the light," says La-Verne. "For they already know the way."

"La-Verne is known for her gently probing style of questioning that allows her to get to the root of the issue," said Jane Doe. "She does this with the wisdom of someone who sees you in your totality without participating in any pre-planned 'pity parties' you might have scheduled that day."

"La-Verne virtually wills you to see positive qualities in yourself and in your personal journey, and she wins every time," said John Doe. "La-Verne's unique ability to separate issues and organize a person's goals is without measure."

To learn more about La-Verne Parris you may contact her:
lvparris@yahoo.com
Tel: 917-705-5829
Follow La-Verne on Twitter: @LaVerne63

CHAPTER 7

How to be Successful and Still Have a Life!

By Helen M. Thamm, MS, APRN, CPC

Have you ever become a *human doing* and lost yourself in your career? Do you go to bed worrying that you missed handling an important work detail or get up in the morning already exhausted just thinking about everything you need to get accomplished? Has your job become your whole life and you no longer feel any joy from it? If your friends ask you out to dinner, do you decline because you don't have enough energy even to have a little fun? Well, if you have answered "yes" to at least one of these questions, you may need a work/life balance makeover!

Being successful does not have to mean giving up family, friends and fun. It is a balancing act. In fact, people who work harder—and harder—often are shown to be less successful. I jokingly have said: "the more you do, the more you'll do." Often the "reward" for working harder is simply getting more tasks to do. I am not advocating being lazy, unmotivated, or shirking your work. Rather I am encouraging successful people to take time away to sharpen their skills, which can mean taking a work-related class, but out of the office, as well as taking time to smell the proverbial roses. (Personally I like Daisies).

I am also advocating setting limits in an assertive, but positive way when the boss gives you too much work just because you complete projects well and on time, or you may not be the boss's friend. I learned early in life that life really is not fair sometimes. Allowing someone to take advantage of you makes you a volunteer, not a victim. Saying what I call the big assertive word with only two letters, (i.e. "no"), can be hard. This can be especially difficult if you work for a boss who uses the autocratic style of leadership. So standing up for yourself admittedly requires finesse. Not standing up can cause even more problems over time though, by increasing stress. I'm sure many of you have tried "stuffing your feelings" literally with food, but this does not help over time. In fact it just made me fat!

Therefore, I recommend learning assertive behavior for anyone whose issue is having trouble setting limits on the amount of work placed on her shoulders. Overwork can negatively impact a person's quality of life. Like any other negative stress, it can even help lead to chronic medical problems like high blood pressure, diabetes, and low back pain!

How then, can a busy, successful person decide if she is actually living only for her work, or if she might want to rebalance some of her time to include what else really matters to her? A simple exercise can help a person identify if overwork is a problem. Draw a circle. Then using the following eight common priorities a healthy person tries to keep in balance, make each piece the appropriate size to represent the amount of time, using twenty four hours as a total. For example, one of the pieces should be labeled "sleep," and that piece should ideally represent between six and nine hours (considered to be a normal sleep range). These are the eight common priorities, but feel free to use one or more of your own: **sleep, work, exercise, eating, personal care, family time, relaxation, self care.**

This is your "pie" of time-priorities in your life. When you finish the exercise, take a look at how much time is spent on work. If you find it takes up more than ten hours of your day, work time may be out of balance with the rest of your life. People may be surprised by how out of balance the work part of their lives has become. Again, most of us want to be successful. Living only to work unfortunately often makes people less effective in their work roles. Over time it can also affect their health and even cause so much family stress that they may lose the support of those they love. Ultimately, many people who don't take the time to take care of themselves, spend time with people they love, and just have a little fun in life often become irritable and resentful of those who are more balanced. They aren't much fun at work—or to work for!

Once a person has identified that work time has become his whole life, he can choose to make some changes. Just identifying there is an imbalance in a person's life is a big first step. The challenge then is what to do about it?

There are many ways to make a small shift to reclaim someone's life from the workaholic style. You only have to make a small change to start. It might be as simple as taking a short walk after work to "come down" from the stress of the day before going home to the family. It might be making a phone call at lunch to a friend or loved one, just to hear the person's voice, without venting about the stress of what is happening. Sometimes just saying "I love you" to a special person is enough to bring that person back to what might really matter in life in the long run—healthy outside relationships.

Whatever the person chooses as a first step, taking it is what is most important. Continuing to practice that small step daily is second most important. Remember a person does not become a *human doing* in a day, so beginning to be a more balanced human being again takes time and repetition doing something new. As strange as it sounds, most people have trouble trying something new, even if doing it makes them feel a little happier for the moment. Change is scary for just about everyone.

Once a person takes a little step to change her life pattern, it often helps her get the courage to try out other options as well. For example, it was difficult for me to make time to exercise to help combat the stress of my work, and to help me stay at the top of my game by getting into better shape, losing some weight, etc. One of the ways that worked for me was asking a friend to go for walks with me. She reciprocated by asking me to go with her to our hot mineral pools. When I didn't feel like exercising, she would gently use her sense of humor to nudge me a bit. She felt my enthusiasm on days when I was more up for exercise helped her get motivated as well.

Another way to help a person get more motivated to take a small step in the right direction, such as getting at least six hours of sleep, is to look at how much time might be "wasted" on TV or other ways people sometimes use to relax that often aren't re-energizing. I found if I just listened to the headlines of the news, then took my shower and went to bed, at the same time every night, it really helped me get the eight hours I need to feel rested, and alert all day long. I also had some trouble getting to sleep sometimes because I have a really active mind. When it was quiet I often went over what I needed to do the next day, or even what I could have done differently that day, rather than just letting sleep come. The answer for me was doing a combination of Yoga stretching exercises, and listening to a positive message or relaxing CD.

I found that not only was it important to try to balance the time I took in different areas of life, but also asked myself the really tough questions, like what did I value most in order to create a healthy work/life balance, while actually enhancing my performance at work. I asked myself what was most important to me: **success, money, time, family, physical and emotional health or reason for being in this world?** I then took some time to get quiet (I meditate, but just sitting quietly and asking yourself the above question can work well). What was your first priority? If success and money outrank all others as your values, ask yourself how much you enjoy what you are doing. If making money and having more success really makes you happier, without causing too much stress, then just a minor adjustment, like taking time to exercise and relax daily, etc. may be fine to create your own life balance, especially if you are a single person without a family.

If family is really important, but you found you spend very little time with them, then adjusting your "pie" of time might help. And, if your reason for being alive might be more a spiritual one (i.e. the main reason you feel we are here), then adjusting how you view what you are doing, and being fully present in the moment with everything you do, might help you set priorities. Spending time in some spiritual activity such as meditation daily, might also be a small step, especially if you are still asking yourself what might be your unique purpose in this world.

Whether getting more time, spending more time with family, finding a reason for being here on earth, or money/success are most important, it is still imperative to have at least a little time outside of work to just live. I have found a simple technique called "closing the door" at the end of a work day really helped me. I just imagine when I close the door to my office that I am closing the door on all the issues, challenges and stresses of the day, and go home to my three kittie "children." When I am home, I am truly home. When I leave home, I also "close the door" to home issues. Therefore when I am working, I am working, and when I am home, I am truly present at my home. That simple technique has really helped me divide my time effectively. Just imagine, if you didn't spend any time worrying about a work issue when you are home how much more enjoyable the evening could be. And, if you are totally present at work, how much more work you could get done, with less effort.

Here is a recap of the ways discussed that can help a person be both successful in her career and "still have a life."

1. Draw your pie of time. Ask yourself: does it feel balanced to you or have you become a human doing.
2. If you identify an imbalance in the amount of time you

spend, for example, at work, choose to make at least one small modification.

3. Follow up making the small change, which can also motivate you to try another.
4. Engage a "buddy" to help you stay motivated. (Some people find a coach is helpful, as well.)
5. Make a list of your personal values. Ask yourself if your present priorities match your beliefs. If you find your values are not in synchrony with either the amount of time you are spending at work, or watching a lot of TV at home, rather than interacting with family/friends, etc., sometimes just a minor adjustment can help.
6. When you are at work, be mindful and present achieving your work goals, but when you leave work, leave worrying about it at the door, i.e., use the close-the-door technique. Also when you leave home, leave home issues and worries behind.
7. When you have made your small step toward rebalancing your work and life, remember to take a little time to celebrate it before making any further changes.

   That first small step is really a huge one that can help you want to make other time/priority adjustments, but as with any accomplishment, it is really important also to give yourself a little "treat" for achieving it.

I hope some of these suggestions help you better balance your life, increase your success and feeling of well being in general, because YOU ARE WORTH IT!

Contact info:
Helen M. Thamm, MS, APRN, CPC
careerreinventions@rtconnect.net
nursecareersuccess@rtconnect.net

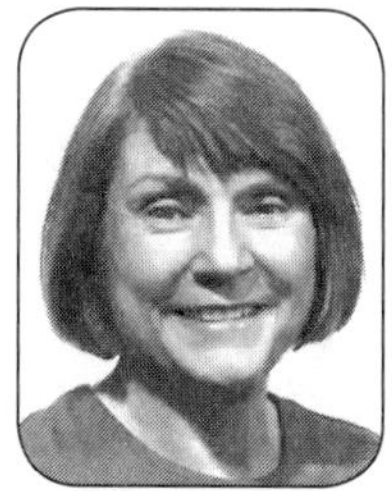
Jeb Schenck, Photographer

About Helen

Helen is a member of the American Nurses' Association and American Psychiatric Nurses' Association, as well as Sigma Theta Tau, the honor society for nursing. Helen then attained certification in Professional Coaching (CPC) as well as Career and Wellness Coaching. She is a graduate of the Career Coach Institute, an ICF (International Coach Federation) approved coaching program. She now specializes in helping nurses and other female professionals succeed more quickly and with less stress as they transition through career stages such as entering management, changing areas of practice, planning for retirement or exploring career options.

She is also a speaker and best-selling author, and is featured as a VIP member of the Cambridge Who's Who Registry. She was interviewed by Elite Radio as an expert in her field. Helen's new managers' success toolkit book *"How to Manage with a Magic Wand, (No, Don't Hit Your 'Problem Employees' Over the Head with It!)"* is available at: helenmthamm.com and popular booksellers. Helen was raised and educated in Chicago, IL, but now lives in beautiful Thermopolis, WY, where she serves her clients throughout the country via telephone coaching and shares success, stress management and life/balance tips at her website and through her tweets (Twitter.com/nursecareersucc).

Contact Info:
Helen Thamm can be reached for questions through her educational website: NurseCareerSuccess.com,
nursecareersuccess@rtconnect.net or
careerreinventions@rtconnect.net

CHAPTER 8

The Best Anti-Aging Secret Ever

By Annie Hodgskiss

How would you like to know a secret to transform your life AND do a body make-over?

And, at the same time you're transforming, you're having so much FUN you won't even realize transformation is happening?

What is this secret?

Ballroom Dancing!

Before you say, "I can't do that," let's dispel the myths and excuses about ballroom dancing right now.

MYTH #1: "I NEED A PARTNER"

I didn't start learning with a partner and I still don't have a consistent partner. I know several people who don't have someone to bring to a dance or to practice with at home. Most dance classes don't require a partner. In fact, you will become a better dancer if you dance with several different people. There are fewer couples in the dance community than you might think. So go to the social dances, take some classes, practice, and have fun. Most people are very sweet and remember what it was like to be a newbie, and they want to help and support you. There will be people to dance with.

MYTH #2: "I HAVE NO RHYTHM"

You can get better with a little bit of practice. Start by tapping to the beat of your own heart. Or have someone help you tap out the beats of songs. Practice does make you better. Remember to have fun. Go to classes or learn at home, and you just might surprise yourself with how much rhythm you do have! If it still bothers you to dance in public, learn to dance at home. You still deserve the healing benefits of dancing!

MYTH #3: "DANCING IS HARD"

There will always be a learning curve to anything new you want to do. Ballroom dancing is no exception; but with every move you make and every class you take, it becomes easier. And it really isn't as hard as you might think. In every beginning class I teach, I start with people who have no idea what a dance move is; after one hour, these same people leave the class dancing. From there it's up to you how much you want to refine each dance.

MYTH #4: "I'M TOO OLD TO LEARN"

I did not grow up dancing. In fact I pretty much grew up doing—nothing. We were poor, without a dad, and with a scared mother. So we did not do or have a lot. I started dancing late in life. You can too. You will find that ballroom dancing keeps you young and gives you energy.

MYTH #5: "I WILL LOOK FUNNY"

I definitely understand the feelings of awkwardness and lack of confidence. Growing up, I developed a very low self-esteem. Actually I didn't have low self-esteem—I just didn't have any at all!

I didn't start out looking good dancing, but it was so much fun, energizing, and such a stress reliever, I kept coming back. Then like anything else, the more I danced the better I became. And you will get better too! Oh, and it helps with self-esteem too – definitely!

Whatever reason you may have not to dance, I encourage you to read on to the end of this chapter to learn all of the benefits you can enjoy when you dance!! The only reason I can think of not to dance is if you prefer to feel old. ☺

Let's get started with why this is the best anti-aging secret I have ever found. It helps you look good and feel good. Ballroom dancing helps REMAKE YOU. It improves your self-esteem, relieves stress, and helps keep your mind revitalized and your body young. It's a great body transformer!

Ok, let's go renew ourselves…

TONE IT

Who would want just to lose weight, when you can lose weight AND transform your body? Why not do both at the same time?

Due to the isometric muscle control that each dance requires, you develop a wonderful tone.

Dancing builds strength by forcing your muscles to resist against your own body weight. This gives you that lean, toned, graceful look.

Imagine every muscle engaged as you move across the floor; movements accentuated by pivots, turns, kicks, sways, bends or rolling-hip motions. Workout intensity and muscles used varies by dance, whether it be waltz, Latin, or swing; but no matter which dance style, each has its own wonderful muscle-toning effect. Plus, every dance helps with coordination, balance, muscle control, and endurance. Dancing is just a lot of fun, so you don't notice that it's exercise and you will, therefore, do it more consistently.

FLEXIBILITY

Stretching is so good for you. When you stretch, you are strengthening and toning because more muscle fibers are being used. Toned muscles help prevent injury, and reduce pain symptoms. Stretching also helps increase energy, improves circulation, and creates a better range of motion for your joints.

Most forms of dance require dancers to perform moves that involve bending and stretching, so dancers naturally become more flexible simply by dancing. The greater the range of motion, the more muscles can flex and extend. [1]

For extra credit ☺ - I would encourage you to stretch frequently throughout your day. Take a minute and stretch. Stretching is vital to your health and staying young.

DANCE FRAME AND CORE

Ballroom dancing helps strengthen your core. Your core or "center" is basically the muscles of the abdomen. Every dance move is initiated by your center. Soon it is second nature to have your core engaged (belly is in and tight) at all times. This encourages strong core muscles, which add strength and stability to your spine and stomach.

Dance frame is imperative to every dance. A good dance frame involves standing tall and proud with enough tone in your torso, arms, and core to be felt by your partner in order to transmit body movements to each other. Frame and core provide a solid foundation for you and your partner to move together. They are also both great posture developers. Standing tall and proud with that dancer posture and your core engaged, can make you look like you just lost 10 pounds! Bring it on! ☺

EXERCISE

We all know we should exercise on a regular basis to enjoy the benefits. It helps manage our weight; and as research shows, prevents high blood pressure, type 2 diabetes, and certain types of cancer— the list goes on.

Dancing is a great workout. It's definitely a sport that will engage all areas of your body and help you lose weight. Just 30 minutes of dancing burns between 200 and 400 calories – the same amount burned by swimming or cycling.[4]

The amount of calories you will burn depends on your body, how vigorously you dance, and the type of dancing you are doing.

It is also great for your heart as stated in the article, *Ballroom Dancers Waltz to Healthier Hearts*, by Allison Aubrey, "Cardiologists are also realizing how powerful dance workouts can be. Italian researchers have found that just 21 minutes of dancing, three times a week, can match the cardiovascular benefits from working out on a treadmill or bicycle."[2] Dancing also gives you the weight-bearing benefits needed to fend off osteoporosis.

If exercise is so good for us, why aren't we all hitting the gym everyday? Does "boring" ring a bell? Wouldn't you rather play than exercise? If you got to play and have fun, how much more regularly would you exercise? Ballroom dancing is a sport, art, and fun all at once. It doesn't feel like exercise and you can do it, at any age, for life.

WILL POWER

If you have a job you dislike, experience trials at home, or face any other daily challenge, your will power is likely depleted by day's end. It makes it harder to do something new; harder to do those things you are supposed to do—like exercise.

A study was conducted with 2 groups of kids. Group A had a great day full of fun activities. Group B had a day of displeasure working on the kids' least favorite subject. The researchers put a bowl of freshly baked cookies on the table and said, "These are not for you, please don't touch." Group A ignored the cookies and talked amongst themselves about the great day they had. Group B squirmed, sat on their hands, moved closer and closer, took a bite and within 10 minutes the cookies were gone. Group B's will power was depleted, and when faced with a challenge, the group gave in and couldn't conquer it. When met with the same challenge, the A's were able to sit contentedly, satisfied with the pleasures of their fun-filled day.[3]

When you've forced yourself to do something all day you don't want to do, it can be difficult to make yourself do yet another chore that you dislike. Your will power has already been depleted.

Exercise is one thing we all acknowledge we need to do, but you don't need to use more will power to do it. Just have fun with your exercise. Dance!

SHAPE UP YOUR MIND

As if all the physical benefits weren't enough, ballroom dancing is also a great brain booster. If you want to keep your mind in shape, you need to work it, just like your body. Dance challenges your mind as well as your muscles.

Dancers need to learn steps and techniques; and coordinate movements with a partner, all to music—these are the types of mental acrobatics that stave off memory loss.

In one study, participants over the age of 75 who engaged in reading, dancing, and playing musical instruments and board games once a week had a 7% lower risk of dementia compared to those who did not. Those who engaged in these activities at least 11 days a month had a 63% lower risk! Wahoo!

Interestingly, of the 11 physical activities considered, only dancing (ballroom dancing, particularly), was tied to a lower dementia risk. Joe Verghese, neurologist at Albert Einstein College of Medicine and a lead researcher of the study, remarked, "This is perhaps because dance music engages the dancer's mind..."

"Dancing may be a triple benefit for the brain. Not only does the physical aspect of dancing increase blood flow to the brain, but also the social aspect of the activity leads to less stress, depression and loneliness. Further, dancing requires memorizing steps and working with a partner, both of which provide mental challenges that are crucial for brain health." [5]

Isn't that exciting? Ballroom dancing can also give you a sexy mind!!

SAFE TOUCH

One of the other wonderful things about ballroom dancing, unlike most other sports or forms of exercise, is the aspect of safe touch. Social inhibitions prevent us from touching, but with ballroom dancing, it comes with the territory. No need for excuses or apologies.

The more and more technologically dependent we become, the further and further away we get from relating with others face-to-face. It's nice to participate in an activity that includes human contact. While you are ballroom dancing, you touch hands, arms, shoulders, backs... all very safe forms of touch. Touch is very healing and something we all crave; we will die physically or emotionally if deprived of it long enough.

It has been documented that babies do not develop or thrive without being cuddled and touched. In some severe instances, the absence of touch has led to death.[6] Touch is essential to our well-being.[7] If we do not receive gentle touch, as we age, we may not die physically; but there is damage done emotionally.

In an interesting study, librarians were instructed to alternate touching and not touching the hands of students as they handed back library cards. When the students were later interviewed, those who had been touched; reported greater positive feelings about themselves, the library, and the librarian than those who had not been touched.[8]

The gentle contact dancing provides naturally releases a hormone in the body, called oxytocin. Oxytocin is a feel-good hormone of calm, love, and healing. It reduces anxiety, helps improve memory, ramps up trust and reduces fear, is associated with friendliness, and reduces anger and aggression. "Under its influence, we see the world and fellow humans in a positive light; we grow; we heal..."—"Lack of touch stunts growth in babies, increases anxiety in all ages, decreases calmness, connectedness, and safety."[10]

Touch helps alleviate stress, pain, anxiety, and reduces depression. Touch can reduce certain stress-inducing hormones like cortisol and releases endorphins in the body to reduce pain and elevate mood.[9] When you are feeling down and someone gives you a hug, don't you feel better? The same feeling of well-being can be provided through the gentle touch of ballroom dance.

WOW!

That's a lot of benefits for one activity!

GET STARTED

Now you MUST be thinking, "How do I get started?"

Introduce yourself to dance. Try out some of my free online dance lessons (www.funfitnessandfood.com). This will help you become more comfortable with some moves before you take a class. You can also practice moves at home anytime you want. And since I emphasize technique, you will get the most health benefits out of each move.

Then, find a beginner class. Places to look are your local parks and rec., community college, social groups, churches, YMCA, and of course, dance studios.

Give them a call; ask if they have any specials or free classes so you can try them out. Ask them what most people wear so you are comfortable.

Finally, sign up and enjoy.

CONTINUE THE TRANSFORMATION

There are many ways you can transform your life with ONE fun activity. You don't have to remember them all because they just happen.

Here are some of the ways Ballroom Dancing can enhance your life:

- Improves heart health
- Boosts memory and prevents dementia
- Relieves stress
- Gives you a sense of well-being
- Is a great aerobic exercise
- Increases strength and endurance
- Improves muscle tone
- Helps prevent osteoporosis
- Improves posture
- Enhances coordination, balance, and poise
- Strengthens core
- Boosts flexibility, agility
- Helps self-confidence
- Cultivates creativity
- Develops body awareness
- Incorporates safe touch
- Helps build social skills
- Improves communication and body language
- Exposes you to the healing of music
- Increases vitality and energy
- Enhances your etiquette and manners
- Allows you to participate in the healing aspects of touch
- Provides a fun and entertaining activity
- Allows your exercise to become a form of play

Try doing all of those things separately. It would take you all day. Dance and all these benefits come with the territory.

So get started!

Get healthy!

Get energized!

Get your own body and mind renewal!!

Bibliography

1. http://www.webmd.com/fitness-exercise/features/dancing-your-way-to-better-health
2. http://www.npr.org/templates/story/story.php?storyId=6622283
3. http://thrivein30.com/lessons/lesson-10_the-mental-health-hat-trick/
4. http://www.livestrong.com/article/339070-ballroom-dance-health-benefits/#ixzz1ZtDGCtho
5. http://en.allexperts.com/q/Aerobics-2267/2009/1/dance-Benefits.htm
6. http://www.transfigurationpittsford.org/Worship/Homilies/Tony/healing_touch.htm
7. http://www.livestrong.com/article/72120-effect-human-contact-newborn-babies/
8. http://library.adoption.com/articles/the-importance-of-touch.html
9. http://www.livestrong.com/article/213200-human-touch-therapy/
10. http://www.dana.org/news/cerebrum/detail.aspx?id=1358,
    The Oxytocin Factor. Kerstin Uvnas Moberg, 2003

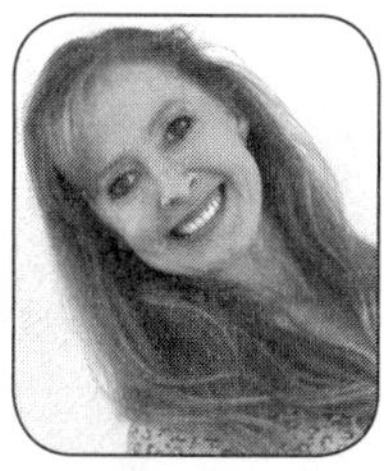

About Annie

Annie Hodgskiss founded her business, Fun Fitness and Food, to help others find the fun and joy in staying fit or getting healthy and fit. Because feeling good should be fun!

She started dancing in 2003, and is now enjoying teaching beginner students the joy of ballroom dancing. Annie is a certified wellness coach and loves to encourage people to eat real food and teach them about the "anti-junk" diet.

Annie, affectionately called Banannie, lives in Central Oregon with her husband Doug.

To get your free online dance lessons, please visit:
www.funfitnessandfood.com

CHAPTER 9

Five Steps to Peak Performance in Sports

By Gavin Kent

How would you like a set of 5 steps, that when followed, and coupled with your physical and sport-specific training, would allow you to achieve your full potential as an athlete? Sounds pretty good, right? The 5 steps that follow will allow you to do just that; reach your FULL potential. They have all been tested over time, and are backed up by multiple sports psychology research studies.

None of the 5 steps have anything to do with physical aspects of training, or diet and nutrition. There are myriads of books discussing those topics. These 5 steps deal exclusively with mental training and conditioning. It is generally accepted that sport is up to 90 percent mental, so shouldn't it follow that the steps to peak performance deal with the mental aspects of preparation and execution?

I start with the premise that has been expressed in ancient Vedic texts, and more recently as a major presupposition of Neural Linguistic Programming (NLP), that we all possess within ourselves everything we need to achieve unlimited success in any undertaking we choose to pursue. Success in sport and almost any other endeavor, begins and ends in the mind. The key is learning to unlock and gain access to these abilities in order to reach our full potential. These 5 steps will help you get started on that path.

STEP ONE: GAIN CONTROL OF YOUR MIND

Step One is "gaining control of your mind" because it must be mastered in order to reach any level of competency in the following steps. Whether it is in the battlefield, the sports arena, or the boardroom, champions are champions because they have learned to control their minds. Winning the internal battle over the mind is a necessary first step in developing an unbeatable mindset.

Without proper training and discipline, the mind is most likely to run wildly, randomly, and unfortunately, often in a self-destructive fashion. The Buddhists have a term for this untamed mind. They call it the "Monkey Mind." A Monkey Mind is characterized as "unsettled; restless; confused; inconsistent; indecisive; uncontrollable." Obviously, these are not helpful traits in developing an unbeatable mindset!

Two great methods for training the untamed mind are breathing exercises and meditation.

Breathing exercises are perhaps the easiest to get started with, and can be done almost anywhere. Belly breathing is often used to calm the mind. The method is easy. Simply sit comfortably with your hands clasped across your belly and concentrate on taking in slow, deep breathes while trying to fill your belly with air. If your hands are rising and falling with each breath, than you are doing it correctly.

Meditation is an excellent method for calming the mind and increasing awareness. It has been used for thousands of years, and is more recently becoming "main stream" as thousands of scientific studies point out both the mental and physical benefits of a consistent meditation practice. Many great books and meditation CDs can be found on Amazon or the various meditation sites on the web.

STEP TWO: GOAL SETTING

This step should be self-evident. There is hardly a self-help or sports performance book on the market that doesn't mention goal setting as a critical part of the process. As crucial as proper goal setting is to peak performance, it is amazing how few athletes and individuals put the time into identifying, committing, acting, and monitoring appropriate goals!

There is no shortage of research studies in sport psychology that support that fact that clear, specific, and dynamic goals clearly improve performance. Goals improve motivation, self-confidence, satisfaction, and pride.

Appropriate goals are goals that are end-result oriented, specific, and achievable. The process should follow these steps:

- Identify a specific goal/outcome
- Create an action plan for goal attainment
- Commit to the action plan
- Work your plan
- Monitor your progress (modify plan or goal as necessary)
- Attain Goal

Be as specific as possible about your goals. Playing well in an upcoming game or event is obviously not a specific goal. Write your goals down and tape or place them in an area where you are sure to see them frequently. This will help keep your commitment level high. You must consistently monitor your progress. This will ensure that you can make modifications to your action plan and/or your goal. Always have a time frame associated with the attainment of your goals.

Have fun with your goal-setting process. Make it a game within your game and you will find your motivation and performance skyrocket!

STEP THREE: VISUALIZATION

Visualization has been utilized by elite athletes for decades. Just watch any Olympic broadcast and you will likely see an athlete mentally rehearsing his or her entire event before the starting gun goes off. What might not be as widely known is that these athletes visualize their performances on a daily (if not several times a day) basis. An athlete is far more likely to achieve a goal if he or she has seen it achieved over and over again in their mind's eye. A slight change to Napoleon Hill's axiom might go… "what the mind can see, the body can achieve."

There is much scientific support for why visualization is so effective. One body of evidence suggests that visualizing certain actions produces the same neurological reactions as performing the physical act would. The mind simply can't tell the difference between something that is vividly imagined and something that is physically occurring.

One way to improve the effectiveness of visualization is to practice it under a state of hypnosis.

Hypnosis isn't some mind control method as old movies and stage hypnotists might suggest. It is merely a relaxed state of focused awareness where the critical reasoning faculty is bypassed. Under this state, positive suggestions and visualizations can go directly into the sub-conscious mind. The sub-conscious mind evaluates these positive suggestions and visualizations as real. Hypnosis is thus a powerful tool for improving the effects of visualization, removing negative beliefs, and reinforcing positive aspects of one's game.

STEP FOUR: RELEASE YOURSELF FROM THE OUTCOME

Releasing yourself from the outcome allows you to play with present moment awareness. Worrying about the outcome increases tension, stress and anxiety; which all adversely affect performance. Outcome thinking takes you out of the "Zone." The

Zone is that state where you are playing with effortless fluidity regardless of what is happening around you. How often have we seen players "choke" under the pressure of the outcome during critical moments of a game?

Obviously, remaining cool, calm and collected while under game pressure is a difficult state to master. However, with consistent work on the first three steps, it will become easier. Simulating this type of pressure during practice sessions will improve performance during actual game/event situations. Just remember to focus on playing your game, and not worrying about the outcome.

STEP FIVE: DEVELOP A MENTAL TOUGHNESS ATTITUDE

Mental toughness is a commonly used term in sports psychology, but it lacks a clear definition. Vince Lombardi, a coach known for instilling an atmosphere of mental toughness, described it as "a disciplined will that refuses to give in. It's a state of mind—you could call it character in action."

Developing a mental toughness attitude involves committing and re-committing to do whatever it takes for you to develop a winner's mindset. Persistence and resilience are necessary. There are sure to be bumps and hurdles to overcome along the way. You need to continue to keep your motivation and focus levels high. Take responsibility for events when appropriate. Don't use excuses.

Mental toughness isn't all about constantly pushing forward as hard as you can. Settling your mind and working on developing calm, focused awareness is a crucial aspect of mental toughness. Wake up with an action plan on how to get better each day. Be flexible enough to change you goals as necessary. This process is dynamic, and takes work.

If you work diligently and persistently on developing the methods and attributes listed in the above five steps there is absolutely no question your performance in all endeavors will improve dramatically. Good Luck!

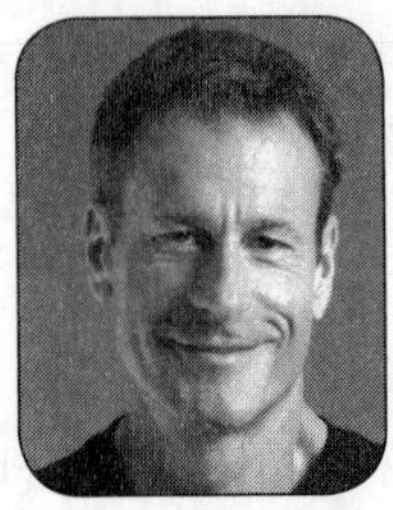

About Gavin

Gavin has been an athlete all his life. After captaining his high school football team, Gavin went on to play rugby for the nationally-renowned rugby team at the University of California, Berkeley, where they won several National Championships. Now a weekend warrior, Gavin has completed several marathons and triathlons. At present, his main passion is an advanced crossfit style workout for "industrial" athletes called Sealfit. Sealfit workouts are designed by former Navy Seals as a method to get ready for the notoriously difficult Navy Seal qualification and training process. These workouts are physically challenging and require a high degree of mental fortitude.

It has always intrigued Gavin how some athletes play above their potential, while others never seem to maximize what they are capable of. He found that the answer lies in the mental aspect of sport. Confidence, playing in the zone, and being that "clutch" player can be learned. It's not only about natural talent. As a result, Gavin has immersed himself in the research and study of the psychology of sport, which has led him to become certified as a Sports Hypnotist.

"I look forward to working with athletes of all ages and capabilities who want achieve their true potential. Unless you work on the mental side of your game, that's just not going to happen. If you do decide to work with me on the mental side of your game, you'll realize the benefits of playing with increased confidence, consistent energy, and perhaps best of all, that feeling of being *in the zone* on demand." ~ Gavin Kent

Other Certifications:
Certified Meditation Instructor. Chopra Center For Wellbeing
Holistic Health Counselor. Institute For Integrative Nutrition
To get started with Gavin call 917-596-7294 or email gkent@athleticperformanceadvantage.com

CHAPTER 10

Eight Tips to Help You Improve and Keep Your Nutritional Habits

By Dexter Tenison

No matter how good your intentions may be, if you don't have the mindset to change or maintain your nutritional habits, it's going to be a bumpy road toward reaching those fitness goals. After all, ask any person who is serious about their health, performance, or physique, and they will tell you that the nutritional component is the key to getting the results you are after. Proper nutritional eating is the foundation to exercise and health. It fuels you when you exercise, causes your body to respond in a positive manner that promotes a faster metabolism, and helps you burn body fat during the huge portions of the day where you are sitting or resting.

Let's say you are finally ready to eat better. You understand the components of a healthy meal, which is eating natural proteins and natural carbohydrates. You even buy some supplements such as fish oils, vitamin D3, and a few others to compliment your successful decision to improve your nutritional situation. This is a great first step! Let me give you some tips to help make sure that you are doing this for the long haul, and not just a short-lived effort that fails once a person's birthday party comes and a piece of fried chicken and cake icing is hanging out of your mouth!

1. FIND THE PEOPLE TO GO TO FOR SUPPORT

Anything that has been done that has been worth doing requires a team greater than yourself. Everything will ultimately go back to you for your nutrition, meaning you are the one feeding yourself. However, the support system you create will allow you to grow in the process and help you overcome obstacles when they occur, and they will! There are various people to consider.

Use your Internet friends. Facebook and other social media sites are huge now and you can have connections from your significant other to your friend who is living abroad 2000 miles away! You will quickly find a group of people who will support your efforts and to whom you can comment about your eating habits. You might even inspire others to eat better as well!

Find a group that shares a common goal as you. Finding a group exercise class or personal fitness trainer that gives great advice, care, and support will go a long way. When you are out of ideas to cook or when you had a bad day and all you want to do is not eat healthy, one of your training partners will pitch in to help you through it. In addition, the exercise session you attended could be just the thing you needed to blow off some steam or redirect your mind.

2. CREATE MEASURABLE BUT REALISTIC NUTRITIONAL GOALS

While being lean, fit, and healthy are great adjectives, they aren't very measurable when a person is trying to establish healthy eating habits. Find the most specific measuring tools you can to establish goals. Do you want to trim the fat off of your thighs or midsection? The scale won't tell you very much about that. However a body fat analysis will because it will divide how much fat you have versus how much lean weight you have. Do you want to eat healthy? A good way to measure is to create a calendar where you can check off specific targets such as making sure you ate a lean protein with vegetables at every meal or minimized the number of times you ate out. Take progress pictures of yourself on a specific day each week or month to see your body changes. Wear a belt and see how many notches you are moving. These tools will keep you on track for healthy eating!

3. RAID THE HOUSE AND WORKPLACE

The environments you are constantly in can make or break you when trying to eat in a healthy manner. If you pass your kitchen where potato chips and cookies (fill in the blank with your weakness) are waiting for you to eat, then chances are they are eventually going to find their way to your mouth. I have a client that has a peer who puts a candy bowl on a table at their workplace. Her peer isn't really triggered by the candy, but my client has a weakness for the sweets. The solution is not a fun one for the frugal person, but the pantries, freezer, kitchen table, and workplace table has to be raided, sent to their proper home, i.e., the trash, and then replaced with better more natural food choices. Cookies made from almond butter would be a great alternative for the kitchen table. Almonds and walnuts can be a great treat to fill the former "candy" now nut, bowl. The freezer now contains healthy meats and veggies to consume. Keep the fridge stocked with fresh veggies and meats you can use to prepare awesome meals.

4. EAT THE HEALTHY FOODS YOU LIKE (NOT THE ONES YOU DON'T)

There is a base level for eating healthy. Most authorities agree on making sure you eat proper amounts of healthy proteins, natural carbohydrates, and healthy fats. The problem is, some people immediately think of the food they hate to eat. For me, it's brussels sprouts. You won't see me eating brussels sprouts any time soon!

The solution is really simple: eat the foods you like and don't eat the foods you dislike. Make a list of the healthy foods you like and then make a list of the foods you don't like. Now, I want you to go one step further. Make a list of foods that your really haven't tried yet, meaning you haven't made a decision if they land in the "like" or "dislike" lists. These lists should be organic, meaning you keep up with it, changing it as you go along. Now, keep to the principles of eating lean proteins, natural carbohydrates, and healthy fats and you should quickly find meals and recipes that follow suit in your likes.

5. CREATE BARRIERS FOR THE WRONG CHOICES

Your current daily habits have created whatever body you are currently wearing. You might need to change parts of your routine or environment to have a healthier, improved eating routine. Do you drive by Ben and Jerry's every day when going home from work and you just have to stop there to get some ice cream? It would be best if you find an alternative route to go home. Your belly size will thank you! For my client I mentioned earlier who has the candy dish on the table, what if she wasn't able to get the dish changed to nuts? A better solution is to avoid the room whenever possible or at least put the candy bowl in a place where they aren't visible. She could even lock them in a filing cabinet! When changing eating habits, convenience is a huge factor in success. Make the good foods convenient and the foods you are trying to avoid very inconvenient to get to. Let's say you are a potato chip junky and you recently threw away the chips from the house. Now that they are gone, the only way you should be able to get chips is to drive to the convenience store, buy the smallest bag, which is going to be at a premium price due to the "convenience" of the store. Most people add barriers for eating better. Switch the situation around and you'll have better success.

6. WHEN LIFE GETS IN THE WAY, BE PREPARED

Cook most of your food on Sunday. Spend a couple of hours cooking foods that you can take to work and can quickly pop into the microwave. You'll know exactly what went into the meal and you won't be worried what ingredients are in the alternative source.

Consider using a frozen meal service. We are finally coming to a day and age where there are companies that offer healthy alternatives of tasty meals that contain only meats, veggies, and snacks. Look for local options first and if there aren't any nearby, search on the Internet.

Have emergency stashes stocked and ready. Sometimes you might not be at a place or in a situation where you can eat. Have alternatives ready. Stash some nuts or another storable healthy snack in a bag in your purse, or have them in your office desk or even your car glove department. This can really get you out of a bind.

7. ASK FRIENDS AND FAMILY TO JOIN IN ON YOUR EFFORTS

One of the biggest complaints I get from people about eating healthy is the isolation from friends and family that comes when you are trying to eat better while they are making no effort at all. I suggest you become the leader to ask them to join you in your efforts. They don't have be as committed as you, maybe they can do a healthy lunch with you, which is when you are around them anyway. Another fun thing to do is to create a challenge with friends and family. While some businesses already do weight loss challenges, I urge you to do something like a body fat loss challenge or a chance for drawing a prize if they complete a challenge. This way, you are creating a support group who will share in your efforts. Not bad!

8. BE BETTER, NOT PERFECT

Have you ever had a friend tell you they are going on a diet and they say something like, "I am going to eat nothing but chicken and broccoli the entire time." Not only is this boring and fairly gross, it is a sure way to create a failure due to an impossible nutritional distress.

I suggest you allow yourself to discover the process of eating in a nutritional way that is healthy, promotes proper weight loss, and allows you to do it for the long term. There are so many avenues you can go with eating in a healthy fashion. Cooking healthy can be far from bland and tasteless. Meals can be gourmet meals! There is an area of nutrition where you learn the ingredients of foods and how they affect your body. There is the psychological aspect of how food affects our moods, whether its based on internal or external factors. You can even grow your own food – so you know exactly what you are getting and that it came from your own yard! There are even more avenues of nutrition what you may not have thought about!

With all of this said, I suggest you allow the process of discovery to occur. If you mess up and have some pizza, so what! You are the captain of your own ship and your journey is going to be yours and yours alone. Just remember to get back at it and use the suggestions I presented to help you along the way. A strong support system will create an environment for you that will distract you from the flashy marketing tactics that unhealthy foods use to lure you into their spell. The whole idea of nutrition is to evaluate what you are currently doing and work on improvement. Reevaluate every so often so that you are going up the ladder of 'better,' not the ladder of disease. You'll be glad you did!

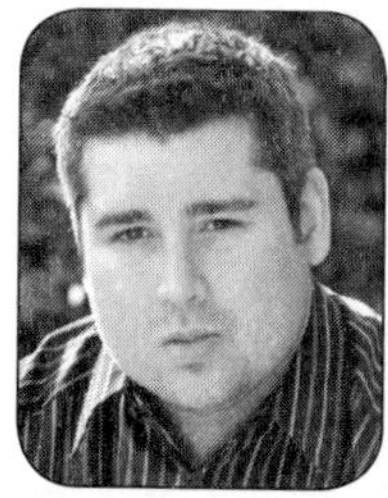

About Dexter

Raised in the small town of Hohenwald located in Middle Tennessee, Dexter Tenison grew up with the same fitness struggles so many Americans face today. With little knowledge of healthy eating and exercise, he struggled with a vicious weight problem throughout childhood and young adulthood. Until he was able to arm himself with proper fitness knowledge and proven healthy-eating techniques, he was unable to beat the unsuccessful yo-yo cycle of pop culture quick-fixes. Once Dexter learned that the keys to long term health and fitness do exist easily within anybody's reach, he couldn't help but share it with the world. It is his passion to help people find their desired destination of becoming more fit and healthy. His aim is to unlock the secrets of health and fitness not just for the people who look good with their shirts off, but for those who never believed it possible. His time tested programs boast 100% success when implemented!

As someone who constantly strives to grow and learn, he sought out his fitness trainer certification with the International Sports Science Association and began working at a gym. He discovered many unethical flaws in the fitness industry that worked against the clients instead of for them. Seeking to find a program that set the highest ethical and educational standards in the industry, Tenison discovered Phil Kaplan's Be Better project. "It's one of the best things I've ever done for my business and my clients," says Tenison. Living by the rule "Be Better," Tenison practices what he preaches. "The goal is not to be perfect it's just consistent improvement. Be better." With this goal Tenison finished his Master's degree in Sports Science graduating with highest honors from the United States Sports Academy. He opened Dexter Tenison Fitness, Inc. and owns Memphis Adventure Boot Camp for Memphians to get outstanding results.

Through his knowledge, personal trial-and-error and deep-rooted passion to help others, Tenison has developed systems with an unequaled 100% success rate when they are applied! "Every one of my clients achieves noticeable results," smiles Tenison. Working with many people who are not comfortable going to a gym where others might judge them or are unsure of their own abilities, he has helped transform his clients into the people they want to be. Humble about his success, Tenison takes joy in seeing his clients' triumph. He has helped people reduce medications, reverse diabetes and overcome cancer, as well as lose weight and gain strength. "People tell me I have changed their lives and I'm in awe of that," says Tenison.

CHAPTER 11

7 Steps To Thrive

By Camille Scielzi

When you woke up this morning, what did you have to say about today? Did you wake up with that feeling of, "Yes, It is going to be a GREAT day!" or one of, "Aaargh, it's another day!" ?? Maybe you were somewhere in between: parts of today were going to be okay and other parts you hoped just to survive.

Your first impression of today is most likely how the day unfolded for you. If you expected a great day, it was. If you expected a bad day, it was. If you just wanted to survive the day, you did. This example demonstrates how powerful our minds truly are: what we think becomes a rooted reality.

We aren't even aware we have set up these mindset scenarios that run our lives every moment of the day. They play like a hidden radio station in the backs of our minds. The lyrics of the songs are based on years of our personal living experiences to which we give some sort of significance and meaning.

What if you don't like the genre of this current playlist? Can you create a new soundtrack for all, or parts, of your life?

Of course you can! Is it my privilege as a life, wellness and business coach to not only say this is possible, but show you how to make it real for you. If our thoughts become reality, then if we want to see a change, or transformation occur in our lives we need to change, or transform, what we are thinking. In other words, it's time for a mental mindshift.

A mindshift begins by taking the time you need, right now -- even if all you have is one minute -- to become present to your desire to thrive rather than just survive. Begin with the belief you will expend little effort and energy creating your thriving state. Thriving requires simplifying life, not complicating it.

Let's dig into my coaching toolbox and see what we can find that will help you thrive. Here we go: *The Take Action Guru 7 Step Thriving Formula.* I use this coaching technique successfully with myself as well as with clients to tune in and reset the soundtrack to something more joyful and fulfilling.

As a coach, and individual, I believe that you already have the wisdom to know what it is you need to thrive. Somewhere life, or someone, intervened and drew your attention away from pursuing that thriving life. It is time to get it back and these steps will take you there.

The formula will help you identify, gather, and refocus your resources to get back to a natural, organic, thriving state quickly, efficiently and authentically.

Here is the formula followed by the detailed "how-to" steps.

The Take Action Guru 7 Step Thriving Formula

1. Select one area to focus your energy.
2. Visualize and document what thriving looks like.
3. Choose one Commitment Action.
4. Communicate that Commitment Action to another person.
5. Set a deadline and complete your Commitment Action.
6. Acknowledge and celebrate the completion.
7. Return to Step 1, and repeat.

Look familiar? It should: almost every self help book and author promotes a similar list of tasks that they have used to define their success. This is great news! It means a universal law has been demonstrated as effective countless times: consistent action produces results when there is an alignment of purpose, belief, and action.

These seven steps, acted on in order, will create the beliefs you need to establish the behaviors that bring you the success you are seeking. Your belief in the process and your commitment to following the steps faithfully and with full integrity will dictate the end result.

Ready to go? Let's get started. You will want to write down the insights you gain from these steps so have a pen and a piece of paper handy. Alternatively, put them on your favorite electronic doodad so you'll always have your personal Thriving Formula with you.

STEP 1: SELECT ONE AREA TO FOCUS YOUR ENERGY

Why only one? Choosing one area of life to thrive in allows you to experience the full spectrum of that one area deeply and meaningfully now. Thriving is not a superficial process. It is about fully expressing yourself in what is important to you.

Selecting one area to focus on now does not eliminate future opportunities for other areas. It also does not deny that you live on multiple levels of existence. Our super busy 21st Century lives sometimes cause us to forget that we have the ability to choose what we want to be experiencing now.

This first step simply focuses your energy on what you need to make life better right now. What you choose is completely up to you and doesn't come with any pressure of being right or wrong. You always have the freedom to make a new choice if the current one no longer is important, or moves down in priority.

If you aren't sure where to start, consider these top five areas of discontent that a coach addresses:

- Career
- Relationships
- Health
- Finances
- Spirituality

Failure to thrive usually means one of these wellness arenas is misaligned. Think of life as a giant puzzle: each wellness piece needs to fit 'just so' to form a complete picture.

Using your preferred writing tool, list the five areas of wellness from above and then assign each one a number from 1-5 in order of decreasing importance to you. Number 1 is the most important area of life for you and number 5 is still important for living fully, but isn't your first priority.

If writing isn't your preferred learning style, feel free to complete this task using other means you do like. For example:

- Using personal photos of events
- Putting together a musical playlist of favorite songs
- Lining up books on these topics by your favorite authors

Once you have your prioritized list, you need to determine whether there is a missing piece to your puzzle or the pieces are just not in the right place. Go back through your list and next to each category ask: is this piece in the right spot of the My Life puzzle?

If the answer is "No," return to the list and label the missing/malfunctioning piece with an N for No. If your answer is Yes, then place a Y next to the piece. Once you have labeled each area, you will see which areas are not thriving. Don't be alarmed if you have identified more than you would like to see.

Your list could look like:

	PRIORITY TODAY (1-5)	WORKING RIGHT? (Y/N)
CAREER	2	N
RELATIONSHIPS	1	Y
HEALTH	3	N
FINANCES	4	N
SPIRITUALITY	5	Y

If you look at your list and you see all "Yes" answers, then the underlying failure to thrive is not a mindshift about alignment. In this case, it is about changing the quality of what you experiencing. The question to ask is, "What do I want the picture to look like?"

STEP 2: VISUALIZE AND DOCUMENT WHAT THRIVING LOOKS LIKE

Look at your line up of priorities. For Priority #1 write down descriptions of what thriving in that area looks like. This list should include answers to the basics: Who, What, When, Why, and How?

- Who is involved with you?
- What are you specifically doing and what emotions are you feeling?
- When is this action occurring and where?
- Why are you doing this? What do you gain?
- How do you know you've been successful?

Give it a full description drawing on experience, inspiration and imagination using your own words. Make this as vivid as you can. If it is a new arena for you, seek out inspiration by talking with friends and family members, or by looking at magazines or even by meditating.

The objective of this step is to create a clear, multi-dimensional picture of what you want to have. Remember: what we mentally believe, we create through actions. Hence we want to create something we would desire!

Example Description:
I have an effortless loving relationship with my husband where we both feel mutually supported daily in our life goals, and are engaging in rewarding activities together during our time together.

I see us laughing, and being affectionate by holding hands and kissing. When I look into his face I feel love flowing from me into him and feel that reciprocated in his look.

STEP 3: CHOOSE ONE COMMITMENT ACTION

This is the step where most people start to think this process feels like work! And honestly, initially it may feel a bit foreign to go through life doing this process mindfully. However, that is short-lived because, once you master this step, it's like developing a muscle: always there ready to be used.

Once this pivotal step becomes an ingrained skill, you will use it effortlessly. You will not have to think about it, it will just happen. It just takes practice.

Looking at your description of thriving for Priority 1, write down the tasks/actions you need to take to bring that description into your everyday world. Keep this list simple -- no more than five items in the beginning!

Then put these steps into a specific order to complete.

Example: Steps for Description in Step 2

1. *Talk to hubby to set aside a set time to be with him that no one else can book*
2. *Choose an activity we enjoy doing together*
3. *Arrange the details to make this together time go smoothly and without worry*

STEP 4: COMMUNICATE THAT COMMITMENT ACTION TO ANOTHER PERSON

Have you ever noticed that people are reluctant to say what they are REALLY up to? Most of us resist doing this because we're afraid the other person will scrutinize us as we perform and then score what we achieve.

Hence, most people keep their plans SECRET and only roll them out with a flourish of "Ta-Da" if they are successful. If they aren't successful, no one else knows. It is a protective tool most of us have learned for surviving in our given environments.

To thrive, you need to let this fear-based model of goal-setting go. Why?

By keeping your desires to yourself you aren't positively activating all of your brain to achieve your goals. By keeping your goal secret, the only accountability you have is to yourself. By telling trusted others your goal, you activate your subconscious by being accountable to another person. Now your brain is fully engaged in getting what you said you wanted.

In addition, it takes energy to keep secrets. It is more productive to use this energy to create what you really desire.

So go ahead and share your goal with someone you trust by telling them what you want to have and how you are going to get it.

Example: of Communication

I will communicate today with my husband this desire and work out the details of our schedules to set up our together time.

STEP 5: SET A DEADLINE AND COMPLETE YOUR COMMITMENT ACTION

Congratulations! If you have made it to this step you are among the top 10% for performance. Most people do not make it to this step. They give up on going after their dreams and settle for something less, or nothing at all. Thriving takes commitment to succeed.

This is a critical choice point. You know what you need to accomplish, so pick a deadline and then go do it. This may sound simple, but it is what builds the conveyor belt of ongoing success.

If this is the sticking point for you, try journaling, and write/draw/sing what it is you are afraid of if you take this action. Some subconscious fear is holding you back. You don't recognize it because, up to now, you have expressed it through rationalizations, justifications, or procrastination.

When interviewed, many great leaders admit to sharing this common experience: it wasn't that fear wasn't present for them, it's that they chose to act despite the fear.

You know what you need to accomplish, so pick a deadline and then go do it.

Example Deadline:

We will have our date within the next 7 days and have one weekly thereafter.

STEP 6: ACKNOWLEDGE AND CELEBRATE THE COMPLETION

It's done! You're thriving! Take a moment to reflect on what you achieved. Don't score your accomplishment. Rather, look at it as an emotional component of who you are. Enjoy being in that space of feeling good and having what you set out to create. Don't forget to share the experience with your accountability partner so they, too, can celebrate!

Example Celebration:

I am feeling happy to be taking action proactively on something that is of importance to me!

STEP 7: RETURN TO STEP 1, AND REPEAT

Oh, you mean there's more? That depends on what you set as your intention for living your life. If it is to live into that highest, most authentic, most rewarding, most fulfilling life for you and those who matter to you, then yes, it's time to go back to the beginning and start the ride all over again.

Before you start again, however, I have a request: please share details of your transformation journey to thrive. I would like to hear how using this formula felt to you, and by sharing your story, others will benefit. Please take a moment to email me at: camille@takeactionguru.com. We'll all celebrate details of your success story, and any constructive feedback for improvement of the formula is welcomed.

Also, please remember to download the free bonus: *Jumpstart Your Success: 3 Steps to Quick Action* that came with your purchase of the book!

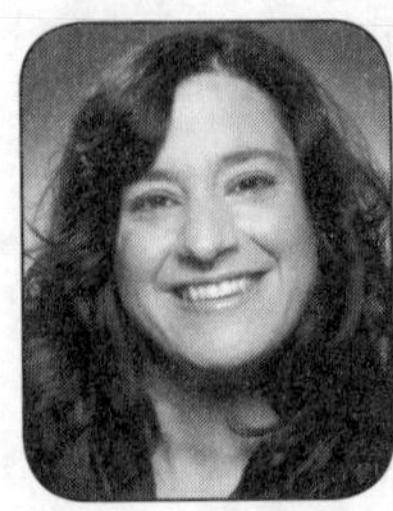

About Camille

Camille Scielzi, the Take Action Guru™, is the founder and certified lead coach of Entrepreneurial Study Hall℠, an online community of holistic health professionals passionate about making a difference in the world. Her mission is to provide the support systems these entrepreneurs need to create an environment where amazing transformations happen naturally for themselves, and those they serve.

Camille coaches these committed professionals to take consistent action to grow sustainable, profitable, and socially responsible businesses. Delivered in a straightforward and often times humorous manner, her advice for building a business that authentically reflects one's personal passion is available weekly through her Internet-based Blog Talk Radio show *Take Action Guru: Small Businesses....Big Missions.....Consistent Action.*

She breaks down the behind-the-scenes details holistic "solopreneurs" are using successfully, and shares them to help all wellness entrepreneurs reach their personal and business goals quickly, efficiently and profitably. Live on-air coaching is an important part of this intimate small business training venue.

As part of the balanced wellness lifestyle she promotes, Camille takes time to rejuvenate and find inspiration. She loves spending time in her home state of New Mexico with her long time spouse Mark. Yoga, Pilates, hiking, reading, cycling and cooking all play an integral part in her physical well-being.

If you would like to know more about Camille's holistic entrepreneurial programs and how they can support you in having amazing wellness transformations, please visit: www.takeactionguru.com.

CHAPTER 12

Two Blood Tests That Can Save Your Life

(and How to Address Two of Your Biggest Heart Health Concerns)

By Inger Pols

I was the kid who ran away from home regularly over vegetables. One time I ran away and decided to hide in the back seat of my parents' car (why not, it was warm and comfy in there!), only to be found sound asleep when they got in to go to the police station to report me missing. My uncle recently remembered my childhood battles with healthy food after seeing a plaque on a restaurant wall featuring John Lennon and his mother. His mother was pleading with John to eat his vegetables, and it read "All I am saying, is give peas a chance."

I didn't know I liked food until I went to a famous French restaurant during graduate school. I even had pea soup and loved it, though since the menu was in French, I didn't realize that was what it was until after I'd eaten it! From there, food and flavor became a focus more than health... until I adopted a four-year old boy from Kazakhstan. Seeing the gruel he ate in the orphanage, it was no surprise he was the size of an 18-month old.

I read that new neural pathways can be built in the brain and learned that most every condition can be reversed or improved through good nutrition. I made it my mission to learn all I could about nutrition and wellness in order to help him make up for his rough start. And so I did.

Then my Dad needed heart surgery and I knew I had to learn more about heart health. At the same time, a friend suffered debilitating side effects from a statin drug, and a fit, healthy neighbor died of a heart attack suddenly in his mid 40s. I had to uncover why 75% of people who have heart attacks have 'normal' cholesterol and why heart attacks occur equally among statin and non-statin users. So I spent hundreds of hours learning what cholesterol is, how it works, and why Total and LDL cholesterol numbers will NOT reflect your true heart-health risk. And now I'd like to share a small part of my discoveries about cholesterol with you.

Our cells need fat and cholesterol to function, but fat and cholesterol can't readily travel through the blood. So the body combines them with protein-covered particles called lipoproteins that can carry a good amount of fat and travel easily through the blood. There are three types of lipoproteins that are particularly important: low-density lipoproteins (LDL), high-density lipoproteins (HDL) and triglycerides.

Low Density Lipoproteins or LDL are responsible for taking the cholesterol from the liver to the body's cells. Once the lipoprotein reaches the cell, the cell attaches to it and extracts the fat and cholesterol it needs.

High-Density Lipoproteins or HDL then take over and play clean up, collecting cholesterol from the bloodstream, LDL and artery walls, and transporting it back to the liver to be recycled. (That's why having higher levels of HDL is a good thing and being HDL deficient can be problem.)

Triglycerides are a type of lipid that is stored in your fat cells. Whenever you eat any extra calories that aren't needed, they are converted into triglycerides. If you need energy between meals, hormones will release them to be burned as fuel. (If that hunger period never arrives because you're eating constantly, that process won't occur and they will remain awaiting their need.)

Triglycerides are an important part of healthy body function; you can't live without them. But like most things, it's about balance; in excess, triglycerides can cause problems. Typically, if your triglycerides are high, you already have or are beginning to develop insulin sensitivity and blood sugar concerns.

We need all three of these transporters in our bodies in order to function. There is no good and bad cholesterol: there is only one cholesterol. LDL and HDL are lipoprotein cholesterol carriers and they are both equally necessary for survival and wellness. LDL has been labeled bad because it can lead to plaque development, but we now know that there are multiple types of LDL.

Research has shown that LDL particles come in different sizes and that large fluffy LDL particles cause no problem. It is the small, dense LDL particles, the smallest of which are called very low density lipoproteins, or VLDLs, that are troublesome. They are tiny enough to squeeze through the lining of the arteries where they can oxidize, or turn rancid, which will cause inflammation. This will begin the process that can ultimately lead to the development of plaque.

If you want an accurate assessment of your heart health, you must get your LDL particle number and size tested. As Dr. Mark Hyman, President of the Institute for Functional Medicine put it,

"Newer tests look at not only the total amount of cholesterol, but the actual size of the cholesterol particles as well as the total number of cholesterol particles. In my view, this is the only test for cholesterol that should be performed. Using older versions of cholesterol testing leads to practicing medicine with blinders on. It is outdated, misleading, and often leads to harmful prescriptions for medications when not indicated. It can also provide a false sense of security when your cholesterol numbers are normal, but the type of cholesterol you have is the small dangerous kind. Studies have found that people with cholesterol level of 300 mg/dl but have very large cholesterol particles have very little risk of cardiovascular disease. On the other hand, people with "normal" cholesterol level such as 150 mg/dl but very small and numerous LDL and HDL cholesterol particles have an extremely high risk of heart disease."

Small LDL are tiny enough to squeeze through the lining of the arteries where they can oxidize, or turn rancid, which will cause inflammation. White blood cells will be dispatched, which is normally a good thing. But if this happens over and over, it can lead to the development of plaque and blood clots. To ensure good heart-health, we need to reduce inflammation and prevent oxidation; the good news is both can be managed through lifestyle changes.

Let's start with what to do if your inflammation is high. You'll know this is the case if you have a C-reactive protein test done.

Chronic low-grade inflammation is a concern even if you have no other heart health markers, because inflammation is shown to exascerbate other health concerns. You can lower inflammation with a statin drug; that is the only real benefit of taking a statin. But the risks have been shown to far outweigh the benefits.

(You might also have heard that statin drugs can lower LDL cholesterol, which is true. But if you have the small, dangerous LDL cholesterol, you will simply have a less of it. Having a little less of it won't significantly reduce your risk of a heart incident; the fact that the small LDL is still present means the risk remains.)

Healthy lifestyle choices such as regular exercise, avoiding processed foods especially trans fats, reducing fructose and managing your blood sugar levels, are all proven anti-inflammatory tactics. Another important factor is balancing your omega 3 and omega 6 fatty acid ratios.

We need both of these essential fatty acids but the problem is that in today's food supply, omega 6 acids are used heavily in processed foods and in restaurants. Vegetable oils such as corn oil, sunflower, soybean, cottonseed and safflower oil contain at least 50% omega 6 and very little omega 3. Corn oil, for example, has a ratio of 60:1 omega 6 to 3, while safflower oil has a ratio of 77:1.

In addition, factory farming reduces the amount of omega 3s in meat, fish, eggs, and vegetables, and increases omega 6 because it is the base of most animal feed, also contributing to the imbalance.

A chicken that is free to eat its normal diet of grass and bugs will lay an egg that is a perfect balance of omega 6 to omega 3. However, the traditional vegetarian grain-fed chicken, (even organic free range), will yield an egg that is more like 20:1 omega 6 to 3. Nature undisturbed knows to work in perfect balance, but our changes in farming have disrupted that balance and left us with an overabundance of omega 6 in our diets.

Ideally, we need a 1:1 ratio of omega 6 to 3, but up to a 4:1 ratio our bodies can still cope fairly well. Unfortunately, the typical American diet is more like a 20:1 up to a 50:1 ratio of 6:3 and that is why it is so important to supplement with or increase consumption of omega 3s. Not only do we need them in isolation for good health, we need them to be in balance with our omega 6 intake. You can assess your omega 3 health through an omega 3 blood test, which I highly recommend even if you already supplement with omega 3s.

There are three types of omega 3 essential fatty acids: ALA, EPA, and DHA.

Two of the three Omega 3s, EPA and DHA, are found in cold water fish like salmon, tuna, herring, cod and mackeral and in seaweed. These are the fatty acids commonly found in omega 3 supplements as well. Because high ALA supplementation has adverse impacts, the third omega 3 has to be ingested through dark green leafy vegetables as well as flax and hemp seeds, and walnuts.

Other anti-inflammatories include polyphenols such as those

found in olive oil and spices such as ginger, cinnamon and tumeric. Studies show that even two teaspoons of spices a day can have a tremendous impact on reducing inflammation. Experimenting with new spices can help reduce your inflammation in a fun and delicious way!

The second concern, LDL oxidation, can be determined directly through LDL oxidation testing or indirectly through LDL particle number and size testing. If your test results show you have the small dense LDL, research indicates that if unaddressed, you will likely have oxidation concerns; it's more a question of when than if.

To reduce LDL oxidation, we need to reduce exposure to free radicals. Free radicals are oxygen atoms deficient in electrons that become reactive in our bodies. They then wander 'freely' through our bodies and cause damage to our tissues and our DNA. Most experts agree that if we could reduce free radical damage, we could slow down the damage that occurs in our bodies as we age.

Antioxidants roam the body as scavengers, looking to prevent cell or tissue damage that leads to disease by donating one of their electrons to neutralize free radicals. Antioxidants are readily found in fruits and vegetables, making getting those 7-13 servings per day even more important.

Vitamin E is a proven defender against oxidation and also helps widen blood vessels and prevent clotting within them. Vitamin E is found in the nuts, seeds and dark green leafy vegetables we know we should eat more of. Vitamin C helps vitamin E return to its active form and helps to combat the free radicals formed by pollution and cigarette smoke.

Nobel prize winner Dr. Linus Pauling believed that vitamin C was essential to heart health. He argued that heart disease is actually a form of chronic scurvy in the body. He discovered that 60% of our ingested vitamin C (we can't make it; we have to eat it) goes to making collagen for the repair of our arteries and cells. Dr.

Pauling recommended 5,000-10,000 IUs a day for optimal health, far above the current 60 IU RDA minimum to avoid scurvy. But recent studies have shown tremendous benefits at a daily dosage of 500 IUs. Because it's water soluble, excess amounts are released, and when that occurs free radicals are carried out too, so we could all benefit from more vitamin C in our diets.

You may have heard about the benefits of coQ10 with respect to reducing free radical production, but it's actually ubiquinol, the active and reduced form of coQ10 (also known as ubiquinone), that provides the benefit. CoQ10 is found in every cell of the body and performs a critical role in cellular energy production and protects against free radical damage. While both ubiquinone and ubiquinol are necessary for sustaining life, more than 90% of the coQ10 found in a healthy person's blood is in the form of ubiquinol.

Our ability to produce coQ10 and then convert it to ubiquinol, even if you eat whole unprocessed foods, diminishes as we age. After age 25, the conversion process becomes more challenging and research shows that taking the reduced form, ubiquinol, has greater health and antioxidant benefits than taking coQ10. Taking ubiquinol can also help you absorb more coQ10 from your food.

In addition to free radical protection and cellular energy, ubiquinol helps manage high blood pressure and benefits seriously ill patients suffering from advanced late-stage congestive heart failure. A study of critically ill patients, each of which had a life expectancy of less than six months, supplemented with ubiquinol for three months. They experienced a 24-50% increase in their heart's ability to pump blood, in some cases tripling their plasma coQ10 levels. They all demonstrated significantly improved heart function by the end of the trial and lived past initial expectations.

Research shows that coQ10 production is significantly reduced on statins so ubiquinol supplementation is a must for anyone taking those drugs.

Oxidation can also occur when unstable vegetable oils are exposed to air or heat.

If you eat out at a restaurant or cook with omega 6 oils, especially at high temperatures, you not only get high omega 6 doses, you increase the likelihood that they will oxidize and turn rancid.

To avoid this, use olive oil only for cold dishes and low-heat cooking. Use butter in moderation and for higher heat, choose grapeseed oil, rice bran oil and coconut oil. Even though we don't care for coconut, my finicky kids enjoy sautéing vegetables in coconut oil. Healthy fats such as coconut oil, olive oil, avocados are antioxidants that help prevent oxidation. And add some garlic: studies have shown it to be a proven reducer of oxidation.

In addition to avoiding vegetable oils exposed to heat and air, we need to avoid trans fats as they lead to LDL oxidation. This unfortunately means reading food labels. And not the marketing language on the front! The American Heart Association recommends no added trans fat consumption beyond what is naturally found in foods, so you have to read the label carefully. Many times I have seen no trans fats advertised, only to read the label and see **partially hydrogenated** or **hydrogenated oils** as ingredients.

Eating a balanced whole food diet, rich in healthy fats, reducing packaged and processed foods, managing blood sugar, and increasing fiber (which helps you manage blood sugar) are heart-health strategies we know about. But there are many more. Reducing trans fats, balancing omega 3 to omega 6 intake, increasing vitamin C and antioxidants, adding ubiquinol along with increasing the use of garlic and spices in your diet are just a few other very important heart-health strategies you can live by.

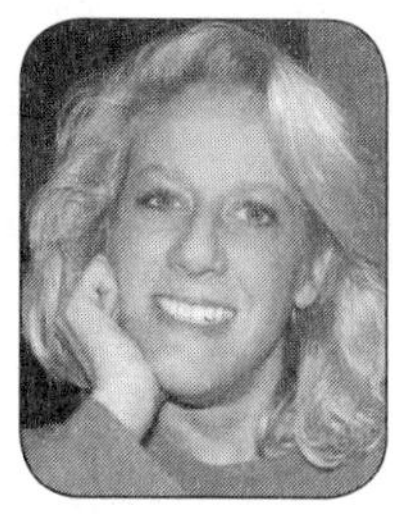

About Inger

After graduating from Yale University and Columbia Business School, Inger Pols spent many years in the corporate world as a Marketing Executive and Consultant. She turned her focus to health and nutrition ten years ago after adopting a four-year old boy from Kazakhstan and a 3-year old girl from Siberia. The size of an 18-month old at age four, her son had little nourishment in utero and in his first four years of life. Inspired by research that virtually everything in the body can be healed and improved through proper nutrition — even new brain synapses can be fired — Inger devoted her life to learning all she could about wellness.

Before becoming a wellness coach, author and speaker, Inger served as director of a renowned online women's wellness company aligned with the clinic founded by Dr. Christiane Northrup. She went back to school to study nutrition and dietary theory and became a Holistic Health Coach and a Stress Management Instructor, a personal trainer, outdoor bootcamp instructor and an indoor cycling coach. Inger served as the Founding Editor of the New England Health Advisory, and wrote an Amazon best-selling e-book called *"What Your Doctor Isn't Telling You – Change Your Life One Bite, One Breath, One Step at a Time."*

Now Inger has created Boot Camps for Life, an online health and wellness company offering audio and video courses to educate and empower you to live a longer, better life. Her first program, Cholesterol and Heart Health Boot Camp, delves deeply into the truth about cholesterol, nutrition and heart-health including what foods really raise your cholesterol, why statins do not prevent a heart attack (they are less effective at reducing your risk than owning a pet) and what you should do instead, and the five essential heart health tests you are most likely not getting — but absolutely should. Covered by insurance, these tests can ensure you avoid a heart attack, stroke, or unnecessary surgery.

Heart disease is the number one cause of death but it can be avoided. And women are not safe; while about 40,000 women will die from breast cancer this year, almost 500,000 women will lose their life to a heart concern. If your cholesterol is high, Inger will show you why. If your cholesterol is normal, she'll share why you may not be safe: 75% of heart attack victims have normal cholesterol. Inger explains it all and then takes you step by step through what you need to do, once you have your test results, to ensure you achieve and maintain long-term heart-health without drugs or surgery.

Inger is available for individual and group coaching, corporate wellness programs, seminars and keynote speeches. She can be reached at: inger@bootcampsforlife.com and offers a free online newsletter and free special reports at: www.ingerpols.com.

CHAPTER 13

Discovering Health Through Adversity

By Sabreena CopeLyn, PhD, ACPEC, SPHR

If you have ever had a doctor stand over your hospital bed and tell you that he's still not sure what you have, but whatever it is, it's killing you; no matter how long ago it was, you remember that moment clearly. For me, I will never forget. It was a fight for my life. I was a young, successful corporate executive with global responsibilities. I worked long hours and traveled a lot, but I loved my job. I was athletic and in good health. Probably one of the last people you would imagine who would have a serious health crisis, but it happened.

Returning to Los Angeles from a long business trip to Europe, I re-packed my suitcase and headed to Texas. During the few days I was home, I felt a little tired and congested, but I didn't think anything about it and continued on my trip to Texas. I attended the meetings on the first day and the dinner that evening. By the next morning, I couldn't get out of bed. Thinking it was just a cold or the flu, I shrugged it off. Each night I thought I would feel better the next morning but I didn't. I stayed in my hotel room bed for five days. I refused the requests to take me to the emergency room because I figured it was just a really bad flu and I'd be feeling better soon. To this day, I still don't know how I drove myself to the airport! By the time I landed in Los Angeles, I could hardly breathe. By time I got to my doctor's office, I could hardly walk. My doctor immediately took a chest x-ray and within a few minutes he had me admitted to the hospital. I had severe pneumonia. That was just the beginning of what played out like an episode of the television show, "House."

While in the hospital being treated for severe pneumonia, I was being triple-dosed on the best antibiotics but my lung kept filling with fluid no matter how many times they drained it. Regardless of what they tried, they couldn't get me over the pneumonia and couldn't figure out why. Then I started coughing up blood clots the size of quarters. Needless to say, the doctors at that point knew that in addition to the severe pneumonia, I also had something else. So they tested me for everything and I mean EVERYTHING! All of the tests came back negative and this left the doctors completely puzzled. By this time all of my vital signs were out of control and I had lost so much blood they had to give me a blood transfusion. Whatever it was, it was rapidly killing me. The doctors then decided to biopsy my lung and sent the sample to the lab. It took the lab an extended period of time to figure out what it was, but the day they finally did figure it out my doctor and the surgeon rushed into my room informing me that I needed to immediately go into surgery. They explained to me that it was a very rare form of bacteria in my lung. They called it a "smart bacteria" because it blocks the blood flow to the organ that it is devouring and killing. That is why the antibiotics weren't working and why I was losing so much blood. So they took me into surgery, removed the part of my lung that they believed had the bacteria and hoped they got it all. And luckily for me, they did. As you can probably imagine, the road to recovery was long and painful. My immune system was completely out of tune and special efforts were required to protect me until it was working properly again.

During my recovery time, I read every book I could get my hands on to understand how and why this happened to me. Why didn't my immune system protect me? The conclusion from all of my research pointed to food choices. I thought I ate healthy but, I realized I was far from it. Do you know that just two tablespoons of refined white sugar can paralyze your immune system for six to eight hours? Do you know how many products you eat and drink everyday that contain substantial amounts of unnatural sugar? I was shocked to see that the food I was eating had little nutritional value and was loaded with many unnatural ingredients that harmed my health. I probably would have gotten more nutrients from eating the box the food came in than the actual food inside the box! Of course I'm joking, but the reality of it was that I spent more time picking out the type of gas I put in my car then I did the food I put in my body. As I continued to learn more about natural health and plant-based nutrition, I transitioned the harmful foods out of my diet and replaced them with organic nutrient-dense plant-based foods. The benefits I have experienced from eating whole plant-based foods are incredible. My health has never been better and I have tons of energy! My immune system is in top working condition. My endurance increased. I lost weight and the dark circles under my eyes vanished. My skin, hair and nails went through an amazing transformation. Furthermore, I can concentrate and focus much longer, thus allowing me to be more productive. I could go on-and-on about the benefits of eating a whole food plant-based diet but you get the picture.

I truly believe my life was spared in order to teach and inspire others who want to improve their health and wellness. I want to share with the world the secrets I discovered during my journey to finding true health. So, several years ago, I took off the "golden hand-cuffs" and left my corporate executive job to start my own business teaching and coaching others how to be smart food consumers and advocates for their own health. I love showing people how great the food tastes and how easy it is to eat healthy. Some people feel they don't have time to make healthy food. My question to them is always; "Do you have time to sit in the doctor's office or be in the hospital?" I can speak from experience, eating healthy is easy. I have been doing this for a long time and I have helped many busy people transition from a Standard

American Diet (SAD) to a whole food plant-based diet. Even small gradual changes can make a significant difference. Despite having a busy schedule, eating healthy must be a top priority. I cannot emphasize this point enough because I understand how easy it is to take your health for granted. That is, until your own health or the health of a loved one is in crisis. That is why I want people to stop digging their own graves with their forks and spoons. Some of you might be saying to yourself; "But I'm pretty healthy already, I don't have any illnesses." Remember, the absence of illness does not equate to health! Here are a few questions to ask yourself.

1. Do you wake up tired in the morning?
2. Do you feel tired after meals?
3. Do you have cravings for junk food?
4. Do you have trouble concentrating and focusing at work?
5. Do you have trouble losing weight and keeping it off?
6. Do you get frequent headaches?
7. Are you frequently congested?
8. Are you frequently constipated?
9. Do you have less than three bowel movements per day?
10. Have you caught a cold virus or the flu more than two times this past year?

A "yes" answer to any of these questions could mean your body is alerting you that your nutrition needs to improve. Mainstream medicine typically does not emphasize the significance of poor nutrition as a major cause of a wide range of health disorders. Although most people are aware of the benefits of good nutrition, the range of conflicting information available to us (the consumer) is often confusing. Therefore, educating people to be smart food consumers and advocates for their own health is my life mission. I want people to see that THEY have the power to transform their own health and I believe the answers are at the grocery store not the drug store.

Including more whole plant-based foods in your diet is helpful to everyone, whether you are dealing with a current health condition or not. Some of you may be worried that you'll have to give up your favorite comfort foods and only eat boring "sticks, seeds, and weeds." I can assure you, even though I eat a plant-based diet that consists of mostly raw (uncooked, unprocessed and unrefined) vegan foods, I still eat all of the "fun" foods. They are just prepared in a different way so that the nutrients remain intact. I make healthy breads, pies, cookies, chocolate, cakes, pizzas, tacos, chips, burgers, pastas, milks, cheeses, ice creams, smoothies, juices, salad dressings, dips, spreads, sauces, and soups. Yes, all of these foods can be made using only plant-based foods. No cooking required!! The food is packed with nutrients, delicious and exciting to eat. Therefore, I want to encourage all of you to proactively invest in your health. Because without your health, nothing else is possible. Learn how to make smart food choices and how to prepare your own healthy food at home. It will save you money and time in the long run. Better yet, do it for the health of it!!

The benefits of consuming a majority of your calories from raw plant-based foods are unarguable. I believe the best health insurance you can have is the food you put in your body. Therefore, always keep a generous supply of fresh fruits, vegetables, herbs, nuts, and seeds in your kitchen. They make easy, satisfying snacks and can also be turned into gourmet delights. In addition to these items, here are a few more favorites that are staples in my kitchen. Many of my clients and students have never heard of these great tasting, nutritionally dense foods so I want to highlight them for you.

1. Kale: one of the most nutrient-dense foods. It is packed with vitamins and minerals. It is getting more and more popular due to recent research pointing out its anti-inflammatory, antioxidant, and anti-cancer nutrients. It has also been praised for its cholesterol-lowering abilities and its ability to help the body detoxify. The secret to loving kale is in the preparation

of it. It's important to destem it and cut the leaves into small pieces. Next, massage the chopped leaves deeply with your hands to soften the kale and give it a cooked texture. Add your other desired salad ingredients, top with a healthy salad dressing and enjoy!

2. Quinoa: (pronounced "Keen-wah") a tiny seed that can be cooked or sprouted. It has a mild nutty flavor and is easy to prepare. It is high in fiber, iron, and protein. It is a complete protein and is much easier for humans to digest than animal meat. Because of that, your body is able to assimilate more of nutrients. Plus, it doesn't have any of the trans fats or saturated fats that animal products have. The best part is after eating quinoa; you will feel full and energized instead of feeling stuffed and sluggish.

3. Shelled Hemp Seed: a small soft seed that has a mild nutty flavor similar to a sunflower seed. It is high in omega 3 and omega 6 essential fatty acids and protein. Like Quinoa, it is also a complete protein. You can eat it right out of the package; sprinkle it on your cereal, non-dairy yogurt, soup, and salads.

4. Nutritional Yeast: thin flakes that have a cheesy flavor. It is very high in all of the B vitamins, including B-12. It is also high in fiber and protein. Sprinkle it on your salads, popcorn, broccoli, soups, and anything else you want.

5. Cacao Powder: (pronounced "Ka-cow") is the bean of the cacao plant and is a natural source of chocolate. It is high in antioxidants, magnesium, fiber, and iron. I make several chocolate raw desserts and smoothies using raw cacao powder. It provides a nice rich chocolate flavor with some nutritional benefits. And it will satisfy your sweet tooth. How great is that!

If any of these items are not available in your local grocery store or health food store, ask the store manager to order it for you or order the item yourself from an online source.

To help get you started on making your own delicious plant-based foods, here are three of my quick and easy recipes. People of all ages love them and they each take less than five minutes to make. Remember, recipes are only guidelines so feel free to adjust the flavors to your liking.

Wholly Guacamole:

Servings: 4

3 avocados, seeded and peeled

½ cup onion, finely diced

3 tablespoons lemon juice

1 teaspoon garlic, crushed

½ teaspoon sea salt

Pinch of cayenne

In a medium bowl, lightly mash the avocados with a fork. Add the remaining ingredients and toss gently to combine. Store the guacamole in an airtight container in the refrigerator for up to three days.

Banana-Cacao (Chocolate) Smoothie:

Servings: 2

1 cup vanilla soy milk
(Silk Very Vanilla brand is recommended)

2 frozen bananas broken into small pieces
(note: always peel bananas before freezing them)

2-3 tablespoons cacao powder
(Navitas Naturals brand is recommended)

Combine all ingredients in a high-power blender. Blend until smooth and creamy. If you want it to be thicker, add more frozen banana. If you want it to be thinner, add more vanilla soy milk.

Cashew Cheese:

Servings: 4

1 cup soaked unsalted and unroasted cashews (soak in water for 2-4 hours and then drain off the water)

1 ½ tablespoons yellow miso

2 tablespoons nutritional yeast (Red Star brand is recommended)

2 tablespoons water (more if needed)

Blend the soaked raw cashews, the nutritional yeast, and the miso in a food processor while adding water a little at a time until the consistency is smooth and creamy. Store the cashew cheese in a sealed container in the refrigerator for up to five days. Cashew cheese tastes great as a sandwich spread and as a dip for vegetables and crackers.

Do you want to lose weight, sleep better, increase your energy and mental clarity, reduce visible signs of aging, build a stronger immune system, and eliminate emotional eating and junk food cravings? Are interested in learning how to add more nutritious, delicious, easy-to-make plant-based foods to your meals? Do you want to explore wellness strategies and get tips for optimizing your health? If so, please visit my website: www.waypointwellness.net. I wish you good health and I'm looking forward to seeing you in one of my classes or working with you in private sessions!

Sabreena CopeLyn, PhD, ACPEC, SPHR

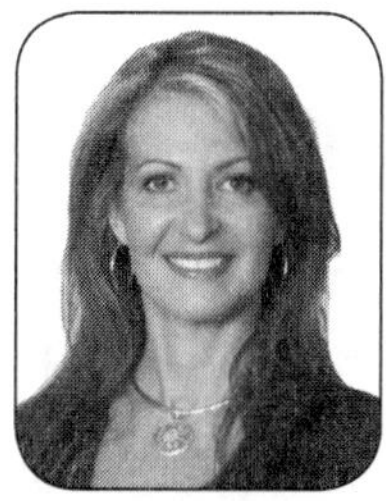

About Sabreena

Dr. Sabreena CopeLyn, PhD, ACPEC, SPHR is a professional speaker, consultant, and coach. She is a leading wellness expert, plant-based nutritionist, and human performance specialist. She has been successfully empowering teams and individuals with advanced strategies designed to enhance human performance for over 20 years. She is the President and Founder of Waypoint Wellness, LLC.

A former international corporate executive and college professor, Dr. CopeLyn understands the challenges of living/working in a fast-paced world and the challenge of staying healthy, focused, and energized. After successfully conquering her own health challenge – which nearly resulted in death – she has dedicated her life to educating others about healthy food choices and optimizing wellness. Using the latest research and cutting-edge solutions in nutrition, psychology, and coaching, she utilizes a unique combination of techniques to deliver extraordinary results for her clients.

Along with providing wellness-education, consultation and coaching, she also teaches clients how to be smart food consumers and how to prepare easy-to-make, nutritious, delicious, gourmet raw/vegan meals at home. Dr. CopeLyn holds Bachelor of Science, Master of Science, and PhD degrees. In addition, she has also achieved over 18 professional certifications, including Dynamic Eating Psychology, Advanced Certified Personal and Executive Coach, Master Weight Loss Coach, Wellness Coach and Instructor, and Certified Gourmet Raw/Vegan Chef and Instructor.

To learn more about Dr. Sabreena CopeLyn and how you can receive free healthy recipes and wellness strategies, visit www.waypointwellness.net.

CHAPTER 14

Facing Life's Challenges – A Holistic Perspective

By Lisa Mercier

As with any life-changing transition in your life, change comes with choice. Most are not easy. Several years ago *Dangerous Minds*, a movie based on a true story was made about a teacher and a class of tough, inner-city teenagers. There was a discussion between a student and the teacher where the student is upset that they are required to go to school and that they are too young to choose otherwise. The instructor reminds them of kids who live in their neighborhood who choose <u>not</u> to get on the bus, but instead skip school, deal drugs and become involved in gangs. In that moment, the class realized that they had, in fact, made a choice. She also implored them to recognize that there were "no victims in this classroom." This exchange really resonated with me. The movie is more than fifteen years old, and I still feel the empowerment of that moment. In spite of how desperate a situation may be, there are always choices.

While change may not always look like a good thing on the surface, we must consider our perception of it and look deeper.

The crossroads in life, and the choices we make, show that we are always growing, moving forward, living! We can transition through these changes, or we can be transformed by them. You always have a choice. You can choose to be a victim of it, or you can take it, learn from it, and emerge a better person on the other side. I truly believe that this applies to all "life transitions" – divorce, death, disease, career change, etc. Those who are successfully navigating these waters are constantly moving. Picture a swimmer in the water, still. What happens? They drown.

Each individual's journey through life is different. However, there are certain commonalities everyone shares. Life brings with it majestic peaks as well as the deepest of valleys. The circumstances may vary, but our lives are all alike in this way. Consider the two following case studies; two women with similar backgrounds were married with two children living in abusive homes. Remember, abuse can take on many forms. While we won't analyze the specific patterns of abuse in each case, know that they exist. Each woman's marriage and lifestyle was devastated by divorce, resulting in extreme financial hardship. While it's never possible to sum up such a drastic life change into a few sentences, we will use this very basic summation for the purpose of this particular example. Although the two women are of like circumstance to this point, this is where the similarities end.

The first woman, Julie, battled her own demons and took on a path of self discovery. She fought to regain control of her finances, took classes and changed jobs. She continuously worked on her emotional and spiritual self, utilized her support network, and stumbled a bit while trying new things. She admits that she's still a "work-in-progress." But, to look at her life now… it is nothing short of a total transformation. Her home is now cheery and full of love, she has a bright future at her new job, and she's helping her kids through their own issues resulting from the divorce. She's independent, hopeful and most importantly, happy.

Diana's is the second story. Diana's life spiraled out of control post-divorce. She turned to alcohol as a means of escape. Initially, it was just a few drinks to take the edge off. However, in an effort to "help," her single friends (also divorced) started taking her out to meet some new people and get her mind off her troubles. Nights out became more frequent and she began actively dating. She ultimately lost her job and was forced to move back in with her parents due to finances. Her ex-husband took her back to court and won custody of their kids, as he was easily able to demonstrate her lack of responsibility and inability to provide a suitable environment for the children.

Two stories that began in a strikingly similar fashion, ended with drastically different results. Although the progression of the two cases happened over the course of several years, it's still shocking how different the circumstances turned out for these two women.

The million dollar question is why and how they ended so differently. Similar women, marital issues, background, environment. Was one woman stronger, more educated, more something? In a nutshell, no. The difference is simple, actually. There aren't any complexities or tricks. I'm sure it's even something you've heard hundreds of times before now. But, let this marinate for a minute.

"IT'S A CHOICE."

It's that simple. We may not have control over life's events during our journey. We do, however, choose how we will react to them, whether or not we will grow, and if we will allow them to destroy us. In short, we choose to be a victim or a survivor.

Some of the world's most inspiring stories are a result of difficult choices made in the face of adversity. Think of those diagnosed with cancer that say, "I'm going to beat this." Bethany Hamilton, the teenage surfer who lost her arm in a shark attack and nearly died, fought the odds to eventually get back in the water. The world rallies around these types of people. Movies are made about their stories. The greater the obstacle, the more amazing the circumstance appears. But when you look closely, did they not make a choice? They chose to be survivors, and to thrive instead of give up. I am humbled by each of these stories, and they never fail to bring me to tears with their courage. However, they are not more significant to the world than Julie, the first woman we looked at. Each one of us has a unique story and special lesson to share. Each person at some point in their life faces a life-altering decision. In fact, we face several over the course of our lifetimes. Births, deaths, marriages, divorces… each brings with it a fork in the road. Life is a series of critical choices.

So how do we make the conscious decision for growth? For decades, science has studied the body's physical aspects and emotional complexities. In recent years, there has been a definite shift in how we view health. Views on health and wellness are coming full circle. We're finally looking at what some cultures have believed for thousands of years. We're beginning to look at not just the biology, but the interaction of the body with its emotional and spiritual counterparts; a "whole self" approach. The growth of alternative and complementary medicine is not a coincidence. People are realizing that health is multi-faceted. Our bodies are incapable of success without the health of our minds, and our minds cannot flourish without the growth of our spirit.

Once we realize that healing must be done from a holistic perspective or by addressing the triad of mind, body and spirit, that's when the real work can begin. By giving each of these aspects of ourselves the respect and action they deserve, we are providing the foundation necessary for growth and strength.

Focusing on these three key areas is important, but it is just as imperative to recognize that healing from life's challenges is a process. There is a progression of stages to be worked through, and some take longer than others. Each person's timeframe is their own. Realize that transitions are a crucial part of our life cycle. Similar to a seed growing unseen beneath the soil, situations both good and bad will occur and bloom. It's important to note that even wonderful changes to our lives, such as a new relationship or the birth of a child, can be very difficult. Our entire outlook shifts, and we experience different experiences we may not have bargained for. How do we navigate these joyous changes, or for that matter, the painful ones?

Preparing for the battle is a war half-won. Commit. Consider. Focus. These are the three basic elements necessary for your journey's foundation.

1. **<u>Commit</u>** – When life is in the middle of an upheaval, it sometimes feels impossible to commit to anything. That's ok. It's normal. If you are only capable of committing to one thing, make sure you are making that commitment to yourself. Commit to nurturing your body, mind and spirit.

Does it sound simplistic? Of course it does. However, you'd be surprised at how often this step is overlooked or discounted. Without a commitment to heal and serve your whole self, it is easy to set aside or fall down the list of priorities. Everyone has busy lives, hectic schedules and things to take care of. More often than not, care for ourselves drops to the bottom of the list. How can you accomplish anything for anyone if you are running on empty? You can't. You have to refill your own cup, so to speak, and your abilities will grow exponentially. Commit to yourself first, and you can serve others in abundance.

Being committed means giving yourself permission to feel all the emotions brought on by a major life change. Squashing anything uncomfortable doesn't allow for the necessary growth and eventual closure to happen. It is easy to blame others and carry bitterness around. But that bitterness results in a black spot in our hearts that keeps us in the past. Giving yourself the 'ok' to be angry or sad is important, as is the knowledge that you will have setbacks. Forgiving yourself the setback enables you to continue moving forward and remain committed.

2. **<u>Consider</u>** – Think about those around you. Who are the five people you are closest to? If you average them out, that is you. Are you surrounding yourself with people who move you forward and cultivate your empower-

ment? Or are they rehashing negativity, gossiping, or otherwise holding you in a painful cycle?

This is a critical concept, and certainly not an easy one to tackle. Now is the time to form your circle of support. It doesn't have to be a large circle. They are your support, your true safety net. It's imperative that this group be filled with those people who will not be judgmental or negative. Now, this isn't a call to go on a friendship-ending crusade. What you are doing is gathering your most trusted relationships to help fuel your transformation. Key life changes call for great strength, and negative energy does nothing to help you through it. You can't afford to remain in a vicious cycle that will hold you back from making the progress you deserve. Don't allow yourself to be surrounded by negativity. It's like a disease… it spreads.

Let your circle know in the very beginning of your journey (even in an email or letter if necessary) how important they are to you. One of the biggest mistakes I see clients make is hiding. Believe me, I get it. I've been there. But hiding under a rock, not calling anyone and wallowing in depression isn't going to help. Trust me. This is why you have a support circle. In your letter, let them know how much you need them. Be very specific when you tell them, "if you don't hear from me for several days, please come looking for me. Come get me, call me, etc. because I very likely won't call you." This is why they are there.

3. **Focus** – Now that you are committed to the process and have surrounded yourself with the right people, it's time to focus. Ask yourself how you are going to put your best foot forward through this change. What does it look like? Address this question in reference to your mind, body and spirit.

This type of goal setting is different for everyone. Admittedly, I am a list maker. More visual people could make a poster board of pictures. Journaling is another option. Whatever works for you! The key is laying a path for yourself to emerge better, stronger. Breaking it down into the three areas helps keep that focus. What steps will you take to nourish your spirit? How will you pursue wellness in your body?

Focus on the physical requirements of this life change. How is this going to affect your finances? Do you need a new budget? Being in control of your money is a lost art, and the people succeeding in this area are doing fine, despite the economy. If necessary find a professional to guide you, but getting a handle on where you are going financially can be an extraordinarily empowering thing.

Perhaps your transition involves your career. Losing a job doesn't have to be the worst thing that ever happened. I know several mid-career people who've been laid off due to the recession. Many of them have entered fields they've always been interested in but never tried, and are happier than ever before. There are many resources out there to help you find your passion. Someone once said to me, "but if I go back to get my degree now, I'll be 50 years old when I graduate!" Aren't you going to be 50 anyway? You can be fifty with a degree or without one. Never let fear hold you back from changing gears if necessary. It could be the best thing you ever do.

When you are focused, it becomes profoundly easier to take action. Start small. Rome wasn't built in a day. If your focus on the body includes more exercise for health and to lose ten pounds, make your goals achievable. Small changes ensure the greatest success. Start by packing your lunch for work instead of eating out. Maybe you cut down a daily trip to Starbucks to twice a week. Walk with a neighbor after dinner. I often recommend yoga and tai chi to my clients because it's enriching both physically and spiritually. You don't need to overhaul your entire life to make small changes that make a difference. Remember that each success, however small, fills your cup a little bit more.

Difficult times in our lives are just that, periods of time. Each one of us will be faced with challenges. Choose to view the challenges as opportunities. It is possible to learn from them and strengthen ourselves. When we use the changes to grow holistically as a person, we not only benefit ourselves but those around us. Invest in yourself. You deserve your time, money and energy. And remember, that you always have a choice. Choose wisely!

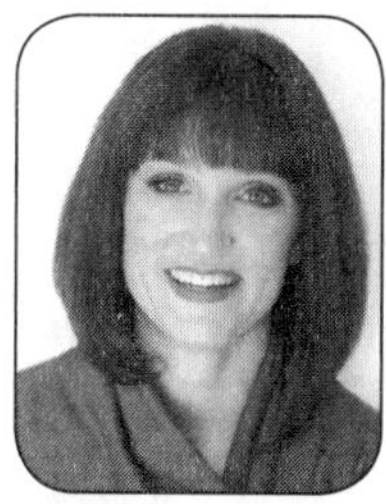

About Lisa

Lisa Mercier is a holistic health advocate, using natural and positive care models to coach others through major life transitions. Her holistic coaching practice changes the lives of clients all over the world by balancing their approach to change with amazing results. Her expertise in grief and divorce recovery resulted in a transformational program helping others work through their issues of anger and sadness to emerge from divorce stronger and happier (www.DivorceToDream.com). Through special engagements and her collection of *Divorce To Dream* books, virtual coaching programs, CD and DVD programs, she provides the ultimate guide to transition through life's challenges with vital energy, a positive outlook, and renewed balance in living. Her three-pronged approach identifies very specific steps to build harmony back into everyday living.

Critically acclaimed as "One of the Best Self-Help Programs Out There," the *"Divorce To Dream"* program is just that, because there is no recovery system out there like it that puts the power of change at your feet and gives you a map for success.

To learn more about Lisa Mercier, the *Divorce To Dream* program, and how you can receive the free Special Report: *"Getting Started: 7 Steps to Creating a Foundation for Change,"* visit: www.DivorceToDream.com or call Toll-Free: 1-(888) 939-HEAL.

CHAPTER 15

Lifestyle Enhancement – Mind and Meditation

For Stress, Pain, Sleep, Memory, Time Management, Productivity, Happiness, and More

By Katrina Luise Everhart, RYT

Meditation, practiced for thousands of years, is still considered new in the US and by most Western medicine practitioners around the world. Yet, more than ten million people practice meditation in the US (Haijtema, 2011). Naysayers, wanting to discredit the effects of meditation, conducted scientific studies only to prove that meditation has positive results, statistically significant positive results. Meditation helps stressed folks sleep, older folks with memory, workers increase productivity, and folks reduce pain and their use of pain medication, whether they have fibromyalgia or cancer.

The mind and the brain are often used interchangeably. Yet, the brain is an organ, while the mind is how we think. It relates to our body, other people, and our environment. Massachusetts General Hospital surprisingly noted that regular meditation causes the cerebral cortex to thicken. The Cortex is the area of the brain that is responsible for higher mental functions. Brain scans of monks who meditate demonstrate that the gray matter of their brains is more than double the size of folks who do not meditate. Why should we care? Often the larger our cortex is, people are able to learn more, have different levels of awareness, have better memory, and some indicate that they are able to manage or control disease.

Like a runner, tennis professional, or Olympian doing drills of some kind, meditation trains our mind. Meditation allows our brain to create new pathways for efficiency. Meditation allows our brain to repair itself. So, like a band-aid that protects a wound, meditation protects our brains from the everyday effects of internal or external stress and damage.

BRAIN WAVES – MEMORY, RECALL, HAPPINESS, DEPRESSION, & PAIN

There are beta, theta, alpha, delta, and gamma brain waves. Beta brain waves occur when we are awake. When we are thinking, most of us are in a beta state. Alpha brain waves occur when we are relaxed. Alpha states help us become creative and learn. Alpha brain waves are believed to help us heal. If we never relax, the stress hormone never goes down and our ability to learn and be creative diminishes. Theta brain waves occur when we are asleep, sometimes known as REM or dream sleep. Theta waves allow us to learn, heal, and grow. Delta waves also occur during sleep or are unconscious. Gamma waves occur when we are hyper-alert and perceptive to our surroundings and information.

One of the changes that meditation can create over time is the emission of more gamma brain waves. Gamma brain waves allow the brain to link or connect information in various locations. That means high gamma-wave activity benefits or increases intelligence, self-control, natural optimistic attitude, and increases compassion. Connections mean we have better memory, more memory capacity, and a higher level to perceive connections between and among systems.

This is particularly helpful for entrepreneurs and anyone who is responsible for product or service delivery, customer service, and/or satisfaction. There is another benefit of gamma brain waves – better recall. If you have ever had trouble remembering a list, a name, a place name, or why you went into a room, *meditation can help you.*

Finally, people with increased gamma waves are less likely to be depressed. In self-reporting surveys, folks report they are more likely to feel they have a fulfilling life. And, there is evidence that meditation also decreases pain by changing the brain waves. Zeidan (2011) noted that four, 20-minute sessions in mindfulness meditation can reduce pain intensity and the unpleasantness folks felt when subjected to painful stimulus.

MEDITATION AND STRESS

Stress increases the levels of cortisol in our bodies. Constant stress over time increases the levels of cortisol, which increases our likelihood of gaining weight, feeling sluggish, fatigued, tired, and unhappy. To combat these items we often turn to food, whether fast-food which has high calorie and fat contents, or comfort foods, which often lead us to overeat.

Cortisol is produced in the cortex of the adrenal glands. It helps us regulate blood pressure and the heart, and it helps us use fats, proteins and glucose; it increases insulin release for blood sugar maintenance, and increases inflammatory responses … or that swelling that occurs in various parts of our bodies, which is not there when we are not stressed. Generally, we have higher cortisol levels in the morning; lower levels in the evening, naturally. By drinking coffee in the morning, we actually increase cortisol in our bodies, above the normally higher levels.

High levels of cortisol tell the body to hold onto fat. High levels also increase blood pressure, suppress thyroid function, impair our cognitive abilities such as thinking, and impair our recall ability. Consistent high levels of cortisol over time can create blood sugar imbalances – which can increase the likelihood of diabetes. Over time, high stress and increased levels of cortisol decrease bone density and our body's ability to heal. That means wounds may stay around longer for someone who has high levels of stress, than for someone with normal cortisol levels. Folks with high levels of stress are also more likely to get colds, the flu, and various other diseases because their immune system is depressed.

High blood pressure is generally a common negative side-effect of stress and high cortisol levels for everyone. Many folks have proposed that various activities beyond meditation do work. For example, going to church is often recommended to reduce stress. Yet, Heinrich, Shoham, Dugas, Kittle & Kurtz, (2011) at Loyola Medicine, note that contrary to earlier studies, religious activity does not help protect against high blood pressure! Meditation does lower blood pressure and thus cortisol levels, which reduce the negative effects.

MEDITATION AND SLEEP

Once we reduce stress and the negative effects of cortisol, we are able to sleep better. Besides calming the mind, meditation helps individuals deal with various sleep disorders. Specifically, meditation helps you focus on the present. While we all have 1,000 thoughts per second, meditation helps train our minds to concentrate or focus on specific things. Contrary to popular belief, we cannot really just empty our minds. We can, however, train them to focus. This focus helps us slow our pulse, which means our blood pressure (BP) falls. As BP decreases, blood supply increases to our extremities, warming our hands and feet, and our brain waves change.

MEDITATION AND PRODUCTIVITY

Stress does not just affect our ability to remember things, sleep, or deal with our health, weight, and general happiness, but it also affects our productivity! "Buck" Montgomery, a believer in the benefits of meditation, instituted a meditation program at his

Detroit chemical manufacturing firm in 1983. At one time 52 workers were meditating 20 minutes before work and 20 minutes in the afternoon on company time. Within three years, "absenteeism fell by 85 percent, productivity rose by 120 percent, injuries dropped by 70 percent, sick days fell by 16 percent—and profit soared by 520 percent. "People enjoyed their work; they were more creative and more productive" as a result of the meditation breaks. Montgomery says. "I tell companies, If you do this, you'll get a return on your investment in one year'" (as quoted by Haijtema, 2011).

Haijtema (2011) quotes a documentary by the Institute for Mindfulness and Management. In the documentary, *Kabat-Zinn* (2008) noted: "You can't stop the waves, but you can surf." Surfing colloquially means that folks are more adaptable and amenable to change and less stressed because they meditate. In India, meditation is common; and in many areas, efficiency and the ability to think creatively is attributed to it. In turn, many believe this makes them successful and more competitive compared with other organizations in countries that do not meditate.

Absenteeism is rampant in the US, but not as prevalent in other countries. Stress alone costs businesses about $300 million a year! Just a one percent reduction, or $3,000,000 is worthwhile for any company to pursue, even if employees are just happier, rested, and less stressed! The latter alone would reduce health insurance premiums and medications.

MEDITATION, TIME, LENGTH, AND TIME MANAGEMENT

Productivity relates to stress, sleep, happiness, and even time-management. The less stress we have and the better sleep we get, the more likely we are to manage our time well. While we can meditate almost anywhere – driving a car or operating any type of power machinery is not a time or place to do so. We can meditate most other places, even in a train station, or on a plane. Time is often a problem. We all have busy lives these days and meditation in the past has been thought by many to be a luxury rather than a necessity. Now, as more people suffer from sleep-deprivation, stress, health, memory, and productivity issues, many are beginning to see it as a necessity.

There are times in which yogic masters believe meditation can be more effective for us – first thing in the morning, between 4 - 8 a.m. and in the late afternoon, early evening between 4 - 8 p.m. Morning is better in most cases when looking just at time and time management. During evening times, we have events whether they are family-related such as music lessons, sports activities, grocery shopping, or just commuting to our home or a business event. But the nice thing to know is that we can meditate anywhere at anytime and it will have benefits. Certainly, a regular time and place helps, but in the current fast-paced world, that is not always feasible. But, meditation always has benefits – even for just three minutes.

Length of meditation is always a concern. Folks often hear about two-and-a–half-hour meditation programs, or one hour meditation classes. While there are meditations that last for hours, there are benefits from three-minute meditations.

Many meditations in Kundalini yoga are done for 11, 22, or 31 minutes. But sessions can be broken down, such as five minutes in the morning and six minutes in the evening, or 15 minutes in the morning and 16 minutes in the evening, or vice-versa. Morning and evening meditations can have different effects. In the morning, meditation can lessen stress and make us more efficient and productive, while evening meditation can calm our bodies and prepare them for sleep. Several medical studies with blood pressure have had participants break up their meditation sessions, similar to how "Buck" Montgomery broke up his company's meditations.

To help you plan for yourself, think about your own schedule and needs, based on time and the results you are seeking. For example, within **three (3)** minutes of meditation, our circulation and blood pressure change. At **five (5)** minutes, our breathing changes. By **11 minutes**, there is a change in our glandular system; our so-called nerves, which create stress and increase cortisol in our bodies, and our cortisol level decreases. In **22 minutes**, the different sides or minds begin to make connections crossing the *corpus callosum* – allowing our different sides, meaning right and left, to connect and heal.

By **31 minutes**, our glands, lungs, blood pressure, and both sides of our mind have synced together. And, if you can possibly meditate **62 minutes** a day, you can change the gray matter of your brain. While 62 minutes may not be feasible, 3, 5, and 11 minutes is doable for most folks – even on a busy schedule. No matter how long you meditate, it is important to remember it takes practice just like running, swimming, tennis, golf, or any other type of sport or hobby. It is better to practice consistently, rather than just one time a week for a long period of time.

HOW TO MEDITATE

Meditation can be done sitting in a chair or on the floor. It is important that if you sit in a chair, it has a straight back so that your spine is straight. If this is not feasible, lying down on a bed, as long as you are not sinking in and you are able to lay straight, will work. Hands can be positioned on your knees with your thumb and forefinger touching, one on top of the other in your lap, or in a specific hand-position or mudra, if you are following a specific meditation style or format, such as Shabad Kriya, nicknamed the Bedtime Meditation. Often the first thing to accomplish is to learn how to breathe deeply from your belly. This alone will benefit your mind and body.

SPECIFIC MEDITATIONS FOR MEMORY AND SLEEP

For **Shabad Kriya,** sit in an easy pose or in a chair with a straight back, place your right hand inside your left, with thumbs touching. Inhale in four equal parts through the nose, much like a sniff, and mentally repeat the words, Sa, Ta, Na, Ma. Hold your breath and mentally repeat the mantra four times, or for 16 counts. Then, exhale in two equal breaths, mentally saying *Wahe Guru. Wahe Guru* means *ecstasy.* And, after you have held your breath, relieving the breath is ecstasy.

Kirtan Kriya, a Kundalini meditation, which also uses the mantra of Sa, Ta, Na, Ma, was used with a Harvard Medical study conducted by Dr. Sat Bir Khalsa. The use of this meditation with mantra demonstrated to help memory within eight weeks time. To do Kirtan Kriya, sit in a straight-backed chair or in an easy pose on the floor. Rest your hands on your knees with your palms up. For each sound, tap one finger to your thumb.

There are many meditations; meditations with mantras or words that are repeated are sometimes difficult to do when others are around, but they can be repeated silently if it is not possible to practice at any other time. These mantras help focus and relax the brain. Just a quick Internet search will yield thousands of results. The best thing to do if you are interested is to determine what you need first, find a meditation or a practitioner to help instruct you, and get started. The nice thing, you do not need any additional equipment and you do not have to go to any special place. You can meditate anywhere, anytime, for less than 15 minutes, and you will achieve benefits.

Remember that Rome was not built in a day, and practicing meditation may not be easy the first few times you try it. Having worked with folks on 11-minute meditations, in the beginning I hear how difficult it is. After a week, I hear it is not so difficult. Within a month, many folks who stick with it cannot imagine not meditating, and after three months, most folks tell me they would rather give up coffee, chocolate, or some other daily ritual than their meditation practice. From personal experience, it is easiest to start with 3 minutes, and start increasing at realistic intervals.

References

Barrett, J. (2011). *Healing Power of Yoga, Yoga Journal.* Retrieved on October 30, 2011 from http://www.yogajournal.com/lifestyle/3016

Boyles, S. (2011). *Zeidan demonstrates Brain Imaging Shows Impact of Brief Mindfulness Meditation Training.* Retrieved October 30, 2011 http://www.webmd.com/balance/news/20110406/meditation-may-reduce-pain

Haijtema, D. (2011). *Management as meditation. Ode Magazine*, Retrieved October 30, 2011 from http://www.odemagazine.com/doc/74/management-as-meditation/

Heinrich, L, Shoham, D. Dugas, L. Kittle, N., Kurtz, A, Lees, B, Rent, S. Richie, W. Stoltenberg, M., Teng, S., Walsh, J., Weaver, M. & Wusu, M. (2011). *Religious activity does not lower blood pressure.* Retrieved October 30, 2011 http://www.loyolamedicine.org/News/News_Releases/news_release_detail.cfm?var_news_release_id=973441444

Rattana, G. (2003). *Shabad Kriya: Bedtime Meditation.* Retrieved on October 30, 2011 from http://www.kundaliniyoga.org/kyt16.html

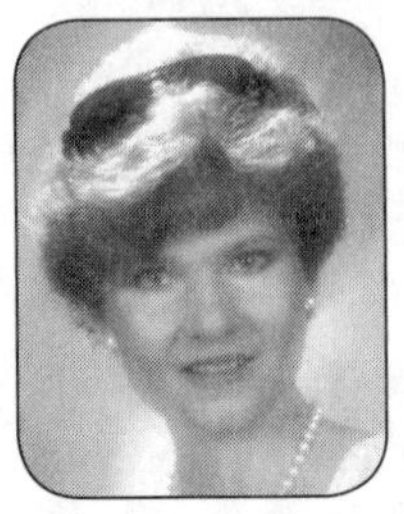

About Katrina

Katrina Everhart grew up in LA. She earned her Bachelor's at Stephens; Masters at University of Missouri, and is ABD at Walden University. Specializing in conflict resolution/mediation, qualitative and quantitative research, systems theory, organizational behavior, project management, competitive intelligence, sea research, integrative medicine, and decision sciences, she's worked in China, Hong Kong, Malaysia, Vietnam, and the US, training and conducting product research, product/service development and marketing.

Past projects include Sprint's DSL, Talking Call Waiting, P&G Floor Care, American Express's Leadership Development. She is an author, artist/weaver (Blackfoot/Navajo styles), 180-year-old-family-farm manager, Certified Project Manager, Indexer, Mediator, Parliamentarian, Researcher, Underwater Naturalist/archaeologist. Her avocations include social entrepreneurship, making buffalo and owl sculptures, yogurt, cheese, knitting, weaving, and crocheting, and helping with genealogical research for heritage societies like DAR and DAC.

Presentations include: *Using Robert's Rules of Order, Native American Justice, Mark Twain, Missouri Indians, Olive VanBibber Boone, Thomas Paine and Common Sense.* She volunteers as a therapeutic clown, scuba dives and racewalks competitively; she is a Barbeque Judge for KCBS, a Registered Yoga Teacher (RYT) in Hatha and Kundalini yoga; is certified in Yoga in Chairs for MS, Reiki Master, Pilates mat, ball, & reformer specialist, Tai Chi, Qigong, and Zumba instructor.

To learn more about Katrina, product development, project management, meditation, and decision sciences to think outside the box, email her at: KatrinaEverhart@yahoo.com or call 573-234-6222.

CHAPTER 16

Truth or Dare

By Warren Martin

I am very appreciative that I have the opportunity to reveal to you my secrets on what has allowed so many of my clients to achieve greatness. The fitness industry has been bombarded with diets, supplements, fitness literature, fitness products, and multiple exercise programs all claiming that they are the answer. The majority of fitness marketing exploits the general population's huge craving for answers to their fitness struggles. Be ready to understand all your misconceptions which were formed by the untruths taught by the fitness industry. Also you will learn how your false perceptions of what should happen, "cause-and-effect," made you fail toward your goals. Then you will be able to design a fail proof plan and know the red flags when shopping for a fitness professional or program so you don't waste money, feel like a failure, or get scammed.

Being in the fitness profession for the last 11 plus years, I've noticed that the fitness industry has been poisoned with untruths for so long that now the consumer is embedded with misconceptions that play into mainstream fitness marketing. Furthermore, I've noticed that individuals false perceptions of what should happen, "cause-and-effect," usually is the root cause of failure either in short term goals or long term maintenance of those goals. Here is the result of this:

- Fitness industry's profits have increased to record highs
- More people are exercising and dieting than ever
- More children and adults are overweight or obese than ever before and their number is still growing
- First time in history that our youth have been faced with getting weight related diseases earlier in life and not expected to outlive their parents

Now is the time to change this trend, so no more turning our cheeks; our kids learn from us responsible grown ups. You have to take charge and learn the truth, learn about yourself, and not let things that sound too good to be true, fool you into empty or short-lived success!

With that said, this will be the most important information you and your trainer will need for your successes with any fitness goal. So let us choose the Truth once and for all and not Dare to choose failure.

1) LEADING UNTRUTHS & MISCONCEPTIONS TOLD BY EXERCISERS AND PROFESSIONALS

*note there are many more but I'm listing some of the top ones I encounter with clients

Food Intake

- Eating healthier will get me to my goals
- Fatty foods or high fat foods make you gain weight
- I have to cut Carbs (breads, sugar, potatoes, etc…) if I want to get to my ultimate goals

Exercise

- Cardio burns off the fat or prevents muscle growth
- This workout style is the best for me to get to my goal

- This exercise will flatten the lower stomach, tone up, or give more peaks to muscle.

2) MY RULES FOR FALSE PERCEPTIONS: THINGS YOU DON'T SAY OR DO

- I just need to cut out the soda or junk
- I'm going to eat smaller portions
- I lost weight this week so I did good
- I gained weight this week because I ate bad Saturday night or ate a cookie
- If I eat too much I'll do extra cardio
- My back or knee or shins or shoulder hurts. I can just work through it because it's nothing
- What are the best Ab exercises to get rid of this belly?

I know every person that is labeled a "Professional" should be trusted but why are so many preaching these statements? Test it out! If a gym guru or a trainer tells you one of the untruths, ask them where the info came from. He or she will not know where they heard it or most likely say it came from "them or they." Who the heck are THEY?

To start off, here is a quick foundation lesson all my clients must know, "The Law of Thermodynamics." To keep it simple, if your energy (Calories in) is lower than your energy (Calories out) then you will lose weight and vice versa. YES it is just that simple! Right now make the decision to use this truth, because it will get you there 100% of the time. My secret is how do I keep you with this concept, mold it to you, and be totally honest with you when it comes to any problems so you can learn from it.

FOOD INTAKE – EXERCISE

Healthy Foods:

Do you agree it is unhealthier to be overweight right now than it is to not eat veggies right now? The leading weight-related diseases are heart disease, stroke, cancer, and diabetes. Do you want a weight-related disease because your weight loss worries are mostly about how healthy a food is, in your eyes? And unfortunately you never end up keeping the weight off and end the life-long yo-yoing that you go through, a friend goes through, or a family member goes through! Yes I promote and encourage healthy eating but the variables that allow fat loss are not as simple as only healthy eating. Look, we are all grown ups, right? You know what is healthy and what is not. How does a fitness professional telling you what food items are healthy help you get to your goals in the big picture? All the successes with hundreds of my clients starts with them understanding these misconceptions and untruths as it relates to them as an individual. Most importantly, it goes back to those basics, the Law of Thermodynamics.

False Perceptions:

"I'm going to eat smaller portions."

Again this is generally good, but everyone's perception of a small, large, or normal portion is different from one person to another. The size of something is all relative to what it is compared to. Your body doesn't store fat because of the volume of food. Remember the Law of Thermodynamics. So it is great if you are going to push your plate away sooner but you must know the calories that you eat no matter what. This way you can make sure you are at the right calorie level to lose fat and now your exercise will be worth it.

Fatty Foods:
FACT: 99.9% of the time when someone fails they put the blame on something that is just not true, whether they know it or not. I already discussed the eating healthier topic, but why are certain foods blamed for making someone fat? This wording is easy to mislead the public because of the word FAT. We hate fat on our bodies and these foods are labeled fatty, so if you don't understand the digestive and energy process then it would sound right that fat would make you fat. This is FALSE! ANY FOOD IS "FATTY" IF TOTAL CALORIES IN A DAY, A

WEEK, A MONTH OR A YEAR IS MORE THAN TOTAL BURNED! Yes fruit is healthier, but if calories from an apple are not used then your body will store it as body fat. All day long, fat is being stored and taken out because the controlling factor is your energy balance at any given moment. How can eating less fatty foods cause some weight loss? Understand that if you stop eating a candy bar and replace it with a fruit then your calories would be reduced by about 150 calories, thus causing weight loss (1lb of fat in about 23 days). That is assuming that those calories are not eventually added back in the day somewhere else. Again the Law trumps fatty foods!

False Perceptions:

"I gained weight this week because I ate unhealthy late Saturday night or I ate a cookie."

Stop with the excuses please. A cookie or an unhealthy meal late at night has never made anyone gain fat. Remember that 'type of food' or 'time of the meal' doesn't make your body store fat. Above I explained that energy is continually being used and stored by the body non-stop. You know what Law I'm taking about by now I hope. If you have gained body fat it is because you ate at a caloric surplus in that given time period. 3500 calories is what it would take for you to gain a pound in a week-that is a 500 caloric surplus every day. That is much more than a cookie!

"I did well this week because I lost weight."

Losing weight does not mean you lost body fat. You must know if you are at a caloric deficit to make the long term results happen. If you lose some weight based on in the scales going down, I promise you will not reach your goal or you will not be able to maintain any results. Have confidence in yourself not the scales!

Carbs are fatty:

Carbs fall into this exact same category. Let me make it simple for you. When you cut out carbs you are cutting out the majority of foods we eat. So guess what happens to your caloric intake? Yes, it is reduced, which will cause weight loss. Doesn't that sound familiar? You have to understand also that if you go into carb depletion your body's fluid levels drop below healthy levels, thus causing a fast weight loss on the scales. Is your goal water loss?? I thought it was fat loss you are looking for? On top of your reduction in calories, your energy levels will also be reduced. This eventually will cause you to eat more again or move less in the day, burning fewer calories and ultimately gaining weight again. So enjoy your carbs and maximize your energy because it is the most important food to allow you to exercise at full potential.

False Perceptions:

"I just need to cut out the soda or bread and I'll be able to reach my goal."

This is great and will help add to the deficit and cut some weight, but it still isn't good enough because you still do not have an understanding of your calorie balance of each day. Over time you will either add calories in other meals or start back consuming them. As I stated earlier, design meal plans that incorporate these bad foods and one that doesn't have them. This way you are making the decision on which to do, but both have you at the right calorie level to reach your goals.

Cardio:

What exercise is known for fat loss? Most likely you said cardio or you have heard a trainer say it. Cardio is very important but it is not the game-maker when it comes to fat loss. Instead of looking at how many hours you did cardio and how much you sweated; look at the grand total amount of calories you burned in a week through cardio. You have to burn 3500 more calories than you consumed in a week to lose 1 pound of fat. So if you did 4 days per week of 30 minute cardio sessions for a beginner to intermediate level, you would burn anywhere from 600 to 1200 calories total. Keeping all other variables constant, you would lose between .18lbs to .34lbs of fat from the cardio. Since cardio doesn't directly burn all your fat off do not think it is ok to not do it. I'm not talking about running only. Cardio comes in many forms because you want to do what burns the most amounts of calories (The Law). So make it fun by using ladders drills, cone drills, circuit training. These are some examples.

False Perceptions:

"If I eat too much I'll do extra cardio"

This thought right off the start tells me that this person feels that exercise can wipe all wrong doing off the table. Cardio most likely can't compensate for eating too much because if you feel that guilty to do extra then the calories are too high. But know how much you overate in calories so you know what to expect for that week with your results.

Type of Workout or Exercises:

I'm frequently asked by people what exercise or workout they need to do to get to their goals and to keep the results this time. I never give the commercialized magic solution they hope I would give. I could make it easy on myself and just say do this and do that and go on my way but my conscience just will not allow it. There is not one exercise or workout that gives life-long results. What does is everything I've talked about in this chapter. You or your trainer need to know how to problem solve but use the facts (L of T) and never use an untruth or a misconception for an excuse or reason why something isn't going right.

Exercise programs are meant to maximize performance in a specific area of fitness. There are many levels so exercise should never get boring or stale. Here are some examples: Flexibility, Balance, Reactive, Strength, Speed, Range of Motion in all planes, Coordination, Power, Endurance and many combinations of all these.

False Perceptions:

"What are the best Ab exercises to get rid of this belly fat?"

To start there are none! I've already talked about what gets rid of body fat, caloric deficit, right? Ab exercises will develop the muscles under that fat layer and help support your back. So do your Ab exercises but if you want to see them, put the main focus on...yes once again your caloric deficit through food intake and high calorie burning exercises.

"My (back or knee or shins or shoulder) hurts. I can just work through it because it's nothing."

Injuries or pains during or after exercise are some of the leading causes of failing an exercise program and eventually gaining weight throughout your life. Any joint pain is your warning. Pains are brought on mostly from dysfunctional movement patterns. So if these issues are not taken care of with corrective exercise then you will probably quit from feeling too much pain, develop an injury and have to stop, or never advance in your abilities which will make exercising stale, boring, or frustrating. You are only as strong as your weakest link.

The Solution:

Here is a simplified list of how to reach your goals (this is general but does need to be specific for each individual):

First, always refer to the Law of Thermodynamics to solve all problems. Do not let false perceptions cause failure.

Second, design your nutrition plan to fit you, convenient foods and what tastes good. Get professional help in finding how many calories you burn and where you need to be at to get to your goal. Then adjust that plan to what allows you to be consistent and is sustainable.

Third, make sure your exercise program is based on improving quality of life and not based off all these untruths and perceptions I've talked about. Practice progressions and a variety of workouts that build all the levels of fitness.

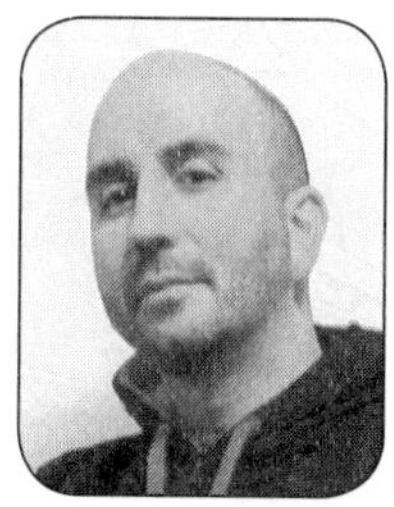

About Warren

Warren Martin has been professionally changing people's lives since 2000. He has always been active and interested in fitness as far back as he can remember. He played all available sports in school and then two days after he graduated from high school he was shipped to Marine Corps Bootcamp, where he was awarded most physically fit in his platoon upon graduation. From there he went on to get his Bachelors in Wellness & Fitness. He then developed his Methods, and WM Fitness has grown to be known as one of the most sound and prominent programs in the nation.

In that Journey, Warren started by learning about the fitness industry through NASM and APEX Fitness Group nutrition, because their foundation was science-based and they were soon to be the leaders in the industry. His programs are used by the normal everyday person up to the Professional Athlete such as an international pro basketball player, top LPGA player, Pro Boxer, and former Mr. Arkansas – bodybuilder, just to name a few.

WWW.WM-FITNESS.COM

Warren's Accomplishments

US Marine Corps
BS Wellness/Fitness Programming Management
Apex Fitness Group - CPT,
NASM-CPT
Reebok Group Fitness & Freemotion Fitness
NSCA member
NASM PES (performance enhancement specialist)
NASM CES (corrective exercise specialist)
HFPN (health fitness provider network)
NESTA-Mixed Martial Arts Conditioning Coach (MMACC)
Specializations: Youth Fitness, Senior Fitness, Weight Management, Fat Loss, Muscle Development, Lower Back Injury, Neck/Shoulder Injury, Foot/Ankle/Knee Injury, Cardio Specialist, SQA performance, Golf performance, Prenatal/Postnatal, and much more.

CHAPTER 17

YOUR PERSONAL 30-DAY WELLNESS CODE

By David Krainiak

I have exciting news for you. Studies show that the progression of even severe heart disease can be reversed by making comprehensive lifestyle changes; so can obesity, early stages of diabetes, cancer, high blood pressure, elevated cholesterol, depression and fatigue. The lifestyle choices we make daily in how we eat, handle stress, activity, and mental thoughts are the greatest underlying contributor to obesity and other chronic physical and mental health conditions.

No matter where you are in your life, I have listed techniques and tips that can benefit anyone – whether you have hit your breaking point, are a disciplined triathlon competitor who is looking for another challenge to test your strength, or someone who just needs to get their mojo back.

After working with thousands of women and studying human excellence, I have noticed distinct traits among the successful and fit clients and the ones that appeared to struggle. Success leaves clues, people who are physically fit and healthy didn't get that way by mistake or by perfect genetics. Is there something you do that you know you are really great at? Maybe its cooking, being an excellent parent, gardening, painting, business, etc. You became great by taking specific action steps. By modeling these actions, you will be on the fast track to your own personal wellness code.

When a NASA ROCKET takes off from Cape Cod Canaveral, it uses up a large portion of its total fuel just to overcome the gravitational pull off the earth. Once it has achieved that, it can virtually coast through space for the rest of the journey.

If the NASA Rocket only used part of its fuel to take off, it wouldn't have gotten far… just like if you take action randomly or just a couple days a week when you're making the effort to jumpstart your personal wellness.

A prevailing personal growth tool that I use is the 30-day trial. It's also a great way to develop new habits because it will ignite your momentum like a rocket taking off, and studies show that it takes about 30 days to create a new habit. In Neuro Linguistic Programming, we refer to taking a long term goal and breaking it down into smaller pieces as a way of "chunking down." It's a lot easier to process and imagine yourself sticking with something for just 30 days than the rest of your life. At the end of the 30 day trial you can always choose to stop if your new habit isn't important to you anymore.

Let's say you want to start a new habit like an exercise program because you want to lose 80 lbs or quit a bad habit like sucking on cancer sticks, because its been 20 years now and deep-down inside you're terrified of the detrimental effects smoking cigarettes may have caused. Thinking about something permanent for the rest of our lives, or a large task like losing 100 pounds, it becomes overwhelming. When we think about the long process involved with our new habit, we all know that getting started and sticking with the new habit for a few weeks is the hard part… Once you've overcome inertia, it's much easier to keep doing. We are always waiting for the perfect time to begin. The perfect time is always right now… there is rarely an ideal time because new events and circumstances always occur.

But what if you thought about making the change only temporarily — say for 30 days — and then you're free to go back to your old habits? That doesn't seem so hard anymore. Exercise daily for just 30 days, then quit if that's what you really want, but after you made it through the hard part, do you really think you will want to quit?

Now if you actually complete a 30-day trial, the rewards are plentiful, including some of these: First, you'll go far enough to establish it as a habit, and it will be easier to maintain this routine than it was to begin it. Secondly, you'll be at the point of breaking an old or creating a new habit at this time. Thirdly, you'll have 30 days of success behind you, which will give you greater confidence that you can continue. And fourthly, you'll gain 30 days worth of achievement, which will give you practical feedback on what you can expect if you continue, putting you in a better place to make informed long-term evaluations and decisions.

Therefore, once you hit the end of the 30-day trial, your ability to make the habit permanent is vastly improved. But even if you aren't ready to make it permanent, you can opt to extend your trial period to 60 or 90 days. The longer you go with the trial period, the easier it will be to lock in the new habit for life. After knowing you made it through the challenging part, it's a lot easier to keep on going.

<u>This 30 day method seems to work best for regular habits.</u> I've had more luck when trying to start a habit that occurs more than just 3 or 4 days a week. However, it can work well if you apply it daily for the first 30 days and then cut back thereafter. This is what I recommend when starting your 30-Day Personal Wellness code.

The dominance of this approach lies in how simplistic it is. Even though doing a certain activity every single day may be less efficient than following a more complicated schedule — a sophisticated weight-training program is a good example because adequate rest is a key component — you'll often be more likely to stick with the daily habit. When you commit to doing something every single day without exception, you can't rationalize or justify missing a day, nor can you promise to make it up later by reshuffling your schedule.

"The journey of a thousand miles begins with a single step"
~ Lao Tzu

Listed below are some of the action steps you could take during the next 30 days as part of your personal wellness code. You can adopt just one, or if you already do many of them, then you could continue to live them and adopt more. I don't suggest that you try to do all of them at once. Remember these action steps are cumulative and are to be adopted over time. Ideally, a habit will be created and eventually become a part of your daily lifestyle.

1. **Take a moment to figure out what you truly want in life.** Most people write down their goals at the beginning of each year and if they are lucky they will review them at the end of the year. Studies show that just writing your goals down one time at the beginning of the year has beneficial results. I suggest you write your top ten goals every single day until you achieve them, and when you do, cross it off the list and add another new one. Many of your ten goals will be the same every day. Don't look at what you wrote previously. The best time to write them down is first thing in the morning and last thing at night right before you go to bed. If you continue this habit past the 30 days, you will be astonished by its impact.

2. **Eat organically**- Organic crops are grown without toxic pesticides or growth hormones. Organic foods have many advantages and it is getting easier to eat organically.

3. **Eat organic fruits and vegetables daily.** The average woman should consume at least 1.5 to 2 cups a day of fruit and 2 to 3 cups of vegetables. The average man should consume at least 2 cups of fruit and 3 cups of vegetables.

4. **Workout every single day** preferably in the morning. Schedule it. We all have the same 24 hours… I have found that training first thing in the morning breeds best results for people. Too many excuses occur before 6:00 pm rolls around, and its time to workout. We call 5:30 am the No Excuse Hour… for most people its just a matter of getting out of bed.

5. **Eliminate sugar and refined foods.** Sugar wreaks havoc on the body.

6. **Drinking a healthy amount of water** is vital to your health. You can never imagine just by drinking a healthy amount of water, you gain tremendous health benefits, and sometimes you can even throw away your migraine medicine or pain killer. Every cell in your body needs water from head to toe. That is why it is so important to drink enough fluid. Hence, next time, if you feel fatigue and headache, it may be the sign of dehydration. Drink at least 8 glasses of water daily. You could carry 8 pennies each day in 1 pocket and every time you drink a glass of water put the penny in the other pocket.

7. **Feed your mind positive info.** Most people eat everyday right? What would happen if you didn't eat for a whole day, a whole week, or a month or two? Most people make a big deal if they miss even a meal because they were so busy. The same way you view feeding your body should be the way you view feeding your brain positive information. Every single day feed your brain positive information . Read a good book even if its for only 15 minutes.

The only disability in life is a bad attitude.
~ Scott Hamilton

8. **Wake up early.** Try waking up at 5:00 am every single day. Imagine how much more you can get done each day.

It is well to be up before daybreak, for such habits contribute to health, wealth, and wisdom. ~ Aristotle

9. **Record everything you eat and drink for the next 30 days.** It is very important to keep a food diary if you are on a diet. It is much more successful with your diet when you do because it would force you to look at what you ate and how much you ate. The National Heart, Lung, and Blood Institute proclaims that "record-keeping is one of the most successful behavioral techniques for weight loss and maintenance." The Harvard School of Public Health says, "It's easy to eat more than you plan to. A daily food intake journal makes you more aware of exactly how much you are eating." You can't improve what you don't record and measure.

10. **Think about all your daily or even life's accomplishments and write them down.** Really go back to that time and think about how excellent you felt when you hit that milestone or accomplished that thing you wanted so badly – that was once just a dream. Record all your accomplishments big and small from the past and present each day. Imagine you will have pages of things to feel great about. Read them often. Remind yourself of how awesome you are. Even if its learning how to cook a new meal or being there for your kids birthday or soccer game, or showing up to all your workouts for the week. Very rarely do people give themselves credit for their accomplishments.

11. **Eliminate drinking any calories** – Stick with water, and organic green tea, no soda, alcohol, fruit juices and sports drinks. This is one of the easiest ways to keep the weight off.

12. **Eat a minimum of 4-6 small balanced meals a day.** Small frequent meals will keep your blood sugar levels stable and keep your energy-level elevated.

13. **Eat Breakfast as soon as you wake up.** One of the best ways to be fat is to skip breakfast and wait until noon to eat.

14. **Exercise every single day** – Exercising daily will make every aspect of your life so much better.

    Did you know if you burn an extra 100 calories daily for 1 year, it will result in a 10 lbs loss, 200 calorie=20 lbs, 300 calories=30 lbs and so on. You can create your own criteria... maybe it a minimum of 30 minutes daily of moderate to intense exercise.

    Lack of activity destroys the good condition of every human being, while movement and methodical physical exercise save it and preserve it. ~ Plato

15. **Join a support team or exercise with others.** In order to stick with the 30-day trial be sure that you meet daily and your team already has a consistent track record of success. You don't want to depend on other people who can't contribute to your success.

16. **Clear the house of junk food.** Keep healthy alternatives for times when you feel you need to cheat. Agree not to buy any high fat or high sugar foods for the next 30 days. That means eliminate all desserts, sweets, soda, fruit juices, candy, chips, etc.

17. **Eliminate TV. Eliminate just 1 hour of TV daily** and that's 40 hours a week over nine 40 hour work weeks. 2 months of additional time. For the next 30 days give up any television. Now if you had an extra 40 hours a week do you think you could find 1 hour a day to work out? Could you learn a new language, learn how to play an instrument, go back to school for a promotion or new career path? Start a new business? Spend more time working on your family or relationships?

18. **Write down 10 things you're grateful for everyday** preferably first thing in the morning or last thing before bed

time. It could be a review of 10 things that you are grateful about for the day. You may just realize that your life is much better then you thought.

19. **Write in your journal daily.** Write for a minimum of 10 minutes daily. Simply record your thoughts. Getting your thought out of your head and onto paper has a liberating effect, try it!

"A life worth living is a life worth recording"

~ Tony Robbins

20. **Meditate Daily.** Agree to meditate for a minimum of ten minutes each day. As you continue to do this, it will be easier to do this longer as your concentration improves. Meditating has hundreds of wonderful benefits that will improve your overall mental and physical health.

All of these principles I have listed are things that can be practiced daily and will be used well with the 30-day trial. If you usually do not adhere to these principles you could do one principle for 30 days, and then after your trial you may find that you love it and it has become something easy for you to adhere to for the past 30 days and is now part of your daily lifestyle. If this is the situation for you, then celebrate your accomplishment then pick another one of these principles. If you're a super-driven type A personality, you may be able to adopt several of these principles daily for the 30-day trial.

The principles I listed are some of the most formidable and possibly life-changing action steps you can merge into your daily life style to enhance your overall personal wellness strategy. Good Luck, and I would love to hear your results!!

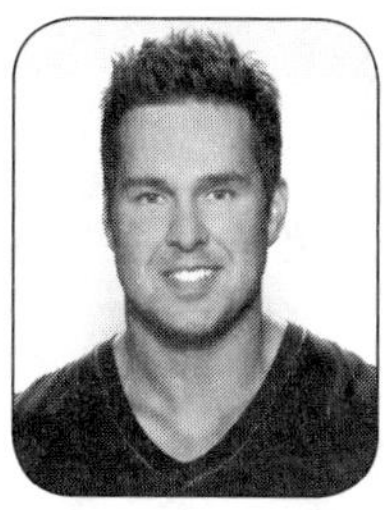

About David

David Krainiak is an entrepreneur, award-winning fitness expert, consultant, actor, and writer. He has appeared in dozens of magazines, newspapers, TV, on the radio, and is available for media opportunities. He has worked on projects from large scale events to building one of the largest women's only boot camp companies in the Midwest with a proven track record of success having helped thousands of women, and is known as the "Go-to-Guy" in women's fitness.

David has taken his years of experience specializing in women's fitness and has "Cracked the fitness and wellness code." David is expanding on a national level with his work of helping women create their dream bodies and the ultimate fitness lifestyle. He also continues as a consultant and works with fitness professionals teaching them how to earn 6-figure incomes and making it to the top of their field.

He can be reached at: David@MIBootCamps.com

CHAPTER 18

Get Your Glow On!

Radiant healthy skin starts from the inside out

By Diane Scarazzini

Wow, what do they do? That is what you think to yourself when you see someone who exudes a radiant glow that shines from every pore. We have all seem them, whether they are a Hollywood star or someone you bump into at a store. The radiant beauty and attractiveness is easy to spot. They must have a secret weapon against growing old and tired like the rest of us. So do they? Probably yes. What I am describing is radiant beauty that gives you a glow. Not the beauty in the artificially, cosmetically altered, made up individual, but the grace, elegance and vitality that oozes from someone who naturally has a glow from a clean internal source. Radiant health always starts from the inside and travels out. No amount of bought creams, lotions, potions, cosmetics can give you this. It can make you look better temporarily.

WHY SKIN AGES AND LOSES ITS YOUTHFUL GLOW

As we age our skin starts to thin, losing collagen and elastin that give it volume, strength and elasticity from hormonal changes, environmental toxins, and free radicals. Blood circulation to the skin diminishes, making less oxygen and nutrients available. The cell membranes of our skin cells become stiff and thick making it harder for nutrients to penetrate the inside. These factors make the skin dull, saggy and wrinkled, the dreaded signs of aging. It is possible to slow or reverse this damage through a nutrient dense diet change, healthy lifestyle alterations and natural product applications to the skin.

TRY AN ELASTICITY (SKIN TURGOR) TEST OF YOUR SKIN TO REVEAL HOW YOU ARE AGING

Pinch the skin on the back of your hand with the thumb and forefinger and hold for five seconds, then release. The shorter the time, the younger the functional age of the skin. Check your results to the table below to see if your skin is functionally younger or older than your biological age (adopted from the Coconut Oil Miracle).

Time (seconds)	Functional Age (years)
1-2	under 30
3-4	30-44
5-9	45-50
10-15	60
35-55	70
56 or more	over 70

SKIN - YOUR BODY'S LARGEST ORGAN

The organs of the body are not all internal. We wear the largest one outside. Our skin covers our entire body. It measures approximately 20 square feet and weighs between 7-9 lbs.

Most people do not give their skin a second thought. It is to them a protective coating that sort of holds everything in. It couldn't be further from the truth. The skin acts as a shield, which insulates against extremes of temperature, damaging sunlight. It manufactures Vitamin D which helps convert calcium into healthy bones. It is such a versatile organ.

The skin cells of your entire body regenerates every 4-5 weeks. The newly created skin cells work their way up to the surface of the skin during this time as an ongoing process. The epidermis is the top layer of skin where you place the creams and other products. The layer beneath the epidermis is the dermis where the collagen and elastin are. The epidermis also has layers, and it is the stratum corneum, the outermost layer where the dead skin cells accumulate. This layer should be exfoliated periodically to reveal the glowing skin you are working for underneath.

YOUR SKIN CAN AND DOES ABSORB CHEMICALS

Though the skin acts as a barrier and shield on the body, it is capable of absorbing toxins. Realize when applying a product to the skin it does not just sit on top. It does get absorbed, with the amount depending how large the molecule is. It is advised to purchase natural products free from harmful chemicals and toxins to use on you face and body. It is said if you can't eat it, don't put it on your skin. Some examples of chemicals that routinely are administered topically via the skin are nicotine patches, hormone therapy, and pain medications. There are some medications that are so toxic, a pregnant woman cannot even touch the tablet.

To show how permeable the skin can be, after rubbing a cut garlic clove on the sole of your foot for about 45 seconds a detection of garlic taste will be in your mouth!

It is a fact of life, when you look good, you feel good. Our skin constantly reflects the internal state of our body. The foods you choose daily become a part of your tissues. You truly are what you eat! The lifestyle choices you make also are very important to getting and maintaining the glow. Here are the eight steps to take to get you on the road to The Glow!

1. LET'S LIGHTEN TOXIC LOADS (IN OUR BODY)

If you counted up the amount of chemicals we are bombarded with daily through ingestion alone, a staggering number of 1000-3000 is usual. By the absorption of the skin alone, the amount between soap, makeup, lotions, perfumes, deodorant is over 500. One moisturizer applied to the face can contain 30 chemicals, and a perfume can contain 400. While it is impossible to completely eliminate toxins and pollutants, we can decrease the amount we are exposed to on a daily basis by taking a few steps.

a. Eat organic food when possible.
If it is too expensive to do this, consider switching to organic instead of the worst offenders of pesticide laden produce called the dirty dozen: grapes (from Chile), cucumbers, spinach, cherries, peaches, cantaloupe (from Mexico), celery, apples, apricots, green beans, strawberries, and bell peppers.

b. Stop Smoking
Tobacco is laden with toxic chemicals, pesticides and pollutants. It causes harmful free radicals to form. The nicotine decreases the blood flow to the skin causing a grayish tone. It also causes the characteristic fine lines and wrinkles around the mouth and face.

c. Limit Alcohol Consumption
Alcohol is very dehydrating, depleting vitamins in the system, and damages the liver, which is vital for detoxing the body. Once the liver is damaged, toxins will accumulate in the body tissues. Alcohol also dilates the blood vessels and capillaries in the skin, and with excess, your face may have a permanent reddish flush.

d. Decrease Caffeine Intake
Caffeine, which is present in coffee, tea, and chocolate, is a toxic, dehydrating and stimulating chemical. It can make the skin prematurely dry and wrinkled.

e. Use Nontoxic Products

The top ten toxic chemicals to avoid in cosmetics are: Parabens which is a preservative (Methyl, Propyl, Butyl, Ethyl), DEA & TEA (foaming agents), Diazolidinyl Urea (preservative), Sodium Lauryl/Laureth Sulfate (harsh detergent), Petrolatum, Propylene Glycol, PVP, VA Copolymer (toxic when inhaled), Sterealkonium Chloride (fabric softner), Synthetic Colors (labeled as FD&C or D&C followed by a number), Synthetic Fragrances (labeled as fragrance). These are found in make-up, lotions, perfumes, shampoos, conditioners, and baby care products.

f. Filter Your Water

Tap water contains many contaminants such as chlorine, fluorides, chemical residues, toxic runoff, and heavy metals. Only pure filtered water should be consumed. A purifying system such as reverse osmosis, distillation, or use of a carbon filter is recommended to clean the water as much as possible.

2. DRINK ENOUGH WATER- A CRITICAL ELEMENT FOR A YOUTHFUL GLOW

The body is made up of 60 -70% water. It is needed for every function of the body. Chronic dehydration is very common today. Excessive consumption of tea, coffee, soda, and juice are to blame. Those drinks cannot be used for the water needed each day, and are dehydrating due to the high sugar and caffeine content.

Water flushes out toxins and wastes from our system, helps with metabolism, and helps our cells stay plumped. It will make the skin show fine lines, wrinkles, thin out and become dull. Even a state of mild dehydration alters your metabolism, cause inflammation, and increases the body's stress hormones.

To tell if you are hydrated enough, your urine output should be fairly frequent with the color of the urine light. If your urine is darker yellow or amber in smaller amounts, you are likely dehydrated.

How Much Water Should I Drink?

A good rule of thumb is to drink half your body weight in ounces spread out daily. For example, if your weight is 120 lbs. 60 ounces of water would be consumed.

3. STRESS LESS

Stress in today's world is unavoidable. The crucial thing is how you react to it. Chronic stress wreaks havoc on all systems of the body causing imbalances including the skin. Remember the jitters of a new job, taking a test, having to perform something that gets you nervous. The result on your face could be hives, a breakout, or one pimple the size of a mountain. The uncontrolled stress caused an imbalance in the delicate hormone levels.

Cortisol is the stress hormone. The substance is always present in the body in varying amounts throughout the day. Cortisol is at the highest level in the morning and lowest a few hours after going to sleep. It does its damage when stress causes a large or continuous release.

As we age cortisol levels increase, rises sharply with stress, and does not return to normal for a much longer time. It has detrimental effects on our skin. It decreases the muscle mass, thins the skin, and makes the blood vessels appear more at the surface of the skin. Collagen and elastin then breaks down prematurely making skin get saggy and lined.

Manage stress with techniques such as deep breathing, meditation, going for a walk, talking to a good friend, warm relaxing bath, writing in a journal, getting enough sleep, or whatever makes you feel better. Your skin will love you for it.

4. MOVE YOUR BODY - MOVE YOUR LYMPH

The lymph system of the body is an elaborate network of lymph vessels, lymph nodes that circulates throughout the entire body. There is twice the amount of lymph fluid as blood. The difference between the blood circulation, and lymph is that lymph flow does not get pumped by the heart.. It is dependent on muscle contractions and movement.. Lymph fluid is vital to drain the body of toxins, wastes, and bacteria. A proper functioning lymph system is crucial for glowing health and vitality. Here is how to keep this system healthy

- Keep adequately hydrated with pure water
- Deep breathing moves lymph fluid
- Avoid constrictive clothing that presses on lymph nodes (underwire bras, very tight garments)
- Get regular exercise- rebounding is great for lymph movement
- Light massage moves lymph and increases lymph flow up to ten times
- Dry skin brushing is invigorating to the skin and encourages lymph movement

5. BRUSH-UP ON DRY SKIN BRUSHING

The skin also known as the third kidney is responsible for detoxification and purging of wastes through the pores. Normally the skin eliminates a pound of toxic waste each day. If the pores are clogged with dead skin cells, the waste will remain in the body, and more burden will be put on the kidneys for elimination. Dry skin brushing rids the dead cells, increases circulation and opens the pores. It has to be done on dry skin prior to a shower or bath. The brush should be natural bristle with a long handle to reach all areas. You will feel invigorated after you shower.

Dry Brush Instruction

- Use gently firm sweeping motion starting at feet, legs, and go upward. Always sweep toward the heart
- Brush your abdomen toward the center
- Brush down the neck, chest
- Brush your hands and upward on your arms
- Brush across top of shoulders & upper back
- Brush lightly around breasts avoiding nipple area

- Facial area can be done with soft brush or dry washcloth
- Shower or bathe

6. GIVE YOURSELF AN OIL CHANGE

Do not be fearful of applying natural oils to the face. Sebum is the oily secretion produced by the skin. Excess is associated with pore clogging, breakouts, and blackheads. Decrease in sebum is associated with dry skin and premature lines and wrinkle formation. It is vital to keep the sebum in balance for radiant glowing flawless skin.

So here is a chemistry fact. Oil dissolves oil. Water cannot dissolve oil unless a detergent is added to it. That is what most OTC cleansers do. This strips skin and causes the sebaceous glands to produce more and more sebum, which can be a problem. It works even on blemished skin to help clean and clear. Simply massage gently into the skin to dissolve out impurities, clean pores and balance the skin. Finish with a warm moist towel to remove. Soft, clean skin awaits you. After cleansing, put a few drops of oil into your hands, rub together, and then gently apply it to your face as a moisturizer. Don't forget the neck and declotage (décolletage) region during the cleansing and moisturizing process.

My Favorite Natural Oils

Coconut

Fresh pressed organic virgin oil solid at room temperature. It will melt on contact in the hands. It is a powerful antioxidant, antibacterial, cleanser, and moisturizer. Used for thousands of years by Polynesian woman known for beautiful skin. Components of coconut oil is similar to sebum. It can be used on entire body.

Jojoba

It technically is not an oil, but liquid wax. A more expensive oil than others, but worth it. It's almost identical to natural sebum. Penetrates the skin, restoring softness, and dissolves clogged pores.

Argan
Named "liquid gold". Versatile for dry and oily skin. Protects against lines, strengthens protein bonds in skin, regulates sebum production. I recommend 100% pure virgin oil.

7. FREE YOURSELF FROM FREE RADICALS - QUENCH THE FIRE

The Root Cause of Aging
The term free radical and damage to the skin and aging are linked. Free radicals are caused every time our cell converts oxygen into energy – which is everyday. We cannot rid ourselves of all free radicals. In normal amounts they actually help get rid of toxins. When the free radicals get to toxic levels through everyday exposure to unhealthy lifestyle and diet, that is, when they rise to toxic levels with no neutralizing or limiting them. The severe damage to our body occurs then.

Free radicals damage the DNA of the cell, and causes havoc in them. Inflammation or "mini fires" are a result of free radical damage, with disease, premature aging, and ultimate destruction of the organs. They can be neutralized by antioxidants. They are a substance capable of slowing or preventing the oxidation and deterioration of other molecules. Some commonly known antioxidants are Vitamin A, C, E and Selenium.

8. ADD SKIN LOVING FOODS TO YOUR DIET

Beautiful, glowing skin starts with a clean, pure healthy body. The foods that are chosen to be consumed fuel the regeneration of the cells in your skin, and the skin also reflects the nutritional quality. Start limiting the amount of animal products, refined, processed, preserved, heavily sugared and salted foods devoid of nutrients from your diet. Start adding organic if possible, enzyme-rich, whole-plant-based foods to your diet such as green leafy and other vegetables and fruits – including berries, legumes, beans, whole grains. Add essential fatty acids to the diet with raw nuts and seeds. Try to eat from the rainbow of colors. Each color of the plant food has its own special phytochemicals that are within it.

SKIN LOVING RECIPES

Smooth Skin

2 large carrots

1 celery stalk

1 apple

1 cucumber

Juice ingredients and drink

Best Lemonade

4 apples

1/2 lemon

Juice and enjoy

Berry Delight

1 cup blackberries

1 cup strawberries

1 cup blueberries

1 cup raspberries

1 apple

Juice ingredients and enjoy

Papaya pudding

1 papaya (scoop out, no seeds)

1 banana

Blend and enjoy

Blend and enjoy

Go Green Pudding

2 ripe mangoes

Green Leaves (small handful of Baby spinach, or Swiss Chard)

Blend and enjoy

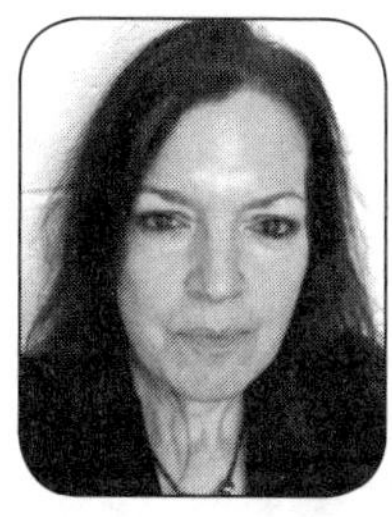

About Diane

Involved in the health and fitness industry for over 30 years, Diane Scarazzini, RN has the experience to empower and guide people to their fullest potential of healthy vibrant living. She lives the lifestyle she teaches, and shows you that can stay youthful and vibrant at any age. As a Registered Professional Nurse with over 30 years clinical experience, she will offer her service as a health and wellness educator, coach, vibrant health mentor, and holistic lifestyle crafter. What sets Diane apart is her background and knowledge in many health areas including nursing, natural health, fitness, nutrition and raw/living foods. Diane is also an N.D. (Traditional Naturopath) and Ph.D in Natural Health, a Certified Raw / Living Food Teacher & Chef. She owned a personal training studio, competed and won multiple bodybuilding competitions.

Diane is a CPT and Boot Camp instructor who owns Feminine Flex Appeal Adventure Boot Camp of Orange County, NY. She is a NYS Licensed Esthetician and natural skin care expert who has worked in the finest spas and holistic centers. Diane presently sees skin care clients in her home. She also holds the distinction of the Certified Professional Coach and Certified Health Coach designations with two impressive coaching institutions. With her, you can clarify your goals, honor your life's mission, and get inspired and motivated to transform your life. She will guide you on a journey to an extraordinary life.

To learn more about Diane Scarazzini and the services she offers,
visit: www.ocnybootcamp.com
or: www.vibranthealthmentor.com
or call 845 496-0322

CHAPTER 19

The Fit Mom Mindset

By Joe Martin

She wakes up every morning, lets the dog out, begins making lunches and breakfasts, starts the coffee, and then begins waking up everyone in the house. Off to school, off to work, and then off to work herself she goes. She works all day, picks up the kids, helps with homework, takes the kids to practices all over town, comes home to make dinner, collapses on the couch for a few hours of mindless TV, and then does it all over again the next day. She is stressed out, tired, overweight, and depressed about how she looks and feels. But she never does a thing about it.

Does this person sound familiar? If you are a mom, chances are it does because SHE is probably YOU. Moms take care of everyone else around them, and then care for themselves last. Their health and happiness suffer, but that's just part of the job of being a mom right? They do it every day and without complaint, but it doesn't have to be that way. If you can't take care of yourself, you can't take care of anyone else. What would happen to your family? What would happen to the rest of your life if you were to get sick? You have to take time out of your day to take care of you. This will not only improve your life, but also the lives of those around you. I'm from Alabama where we have an old saying, "If mama ain't happy, ain't nobody happy." My goal is to get you in the proper mind set to get into the shape you want and deserve to be in. Here are the three steps to follow in order to achieve the Fit Mom Mindset: eliminate the excuses, believe you can do it, and decide whether you are committed or just interested.

Let's look at the real reason you are in the shape you are in now. It is you. I know that sounds harsh, but it is the truth. It's because of ________(insert excuse here).

-injury

-illness

-my schedule

-my family

-job

-genetics

-age

-weather

Any of those sound familiar? The list goes on and on. Sure they didn't help you, but they didn't cause the whole thing. They didn't make you eat all that junk and/or be sedentary for so long. Those are contributing factors; you are the root cause.

I've used a few excuses, so I know. I look back to when I was overweight and it is a wonder I wasn't bigger than I was. Would splitting a 6-pack of donuts, washed down with a Mountain Dew seem like a good idea? Yep. That's what happens when two lineman ride home together after football practice. Then I would eat dinner soon after getting home.

I ate whenever I could and however much I could handle. Sugar, fat, salt, grease? Yes please.

You need to look at yourself and the mirror and realize that it is not something keeping you from getting into better shape and losing weight RIGHT NOW. It is you. The sooner you realize that, the sooner you can fix it.

If you're hurt or sick, are you eating absolutely as clean as you can? Are you working around the injury or illness as best as you can? Did you do all the necessary rehab? Successful surgery without the proper rehab is worthless. If you hurt your upper body, do lower body and core work. If you hurt your lower body, do upper body and core work. The worst thing to be ill or injured is your attitude. Fix your attitude and you will be surprised what you can accomplish.

I'm too busy to exercise! Do you surf the Internet, watch TV, etc…? You have time, go find it. Too busy watching kids? Kids can either watch you workout or join in the fun. My son plays in the garage where I do my workouts on a regular basis. Exercising in front of your kids is great for both of you. It shows your children that mommy sees exercise as a priority, plus you get your workout in.

Do you have bad genetics? That can be tough and there is nothing you can do about genetics. What you can do is bust your hump to overcome it. You may not have it as easy as some people, but that shouldn't stop you from trying. The worst reason in the world not to do something is because it is hard.

Do you think you're too old? Not too old to do SOMETHING. Your pace may not be as rigorous as it was back in the day, but if you have a pulse you can still have some kind of pace. A little bit of something always beats a whole lot of nothing.

It's too cold/rainy/hot to exercise and you don't like to exercise indoors. Learn to dress for the weather or learn to like exercising indoors. Simple as that. Every workout may not be ideal, but neither is being overweight and out of shape.

I'm saying all this for 2 reasons.

-I've been there

-I care.

I want you all to be successful, healthy, and happy. So look deep within and have an honest look at yourself. Before you go blaming the world for the situation you're in, decide what you can do to fix it.

The majority of people in life are held back because they have crippling self doubt. They are afraid to try new things because there is a chance they will fail and they cannot afford to take that chance. I'm pretty good at recognizing it because it has held me back from reaching my goals too.

You're talking to a guy who started a boot camp for women at 5:30 am in a parking lot in the middle of a terrible recession. You think I didn't have a few doubts? Several times in the days leading up to the start of camp, I would picture myself teaching tumbleweeds how to do pushups.

But I had two things that convinced me I could do it. One, I knew others had done it before and had been successful. Two, I knew in my heart this was something I would be good at. I think back on my first camp and I compare them to the first people who drank milk. Sure it looks easy now, but would you have wanted to be the first one? Drink what? Out of where?

Have you ever heard of Roger Bannister? He was the first man to ever run a mile under 4 minutes. Before he accomplished that, people (even scientists) thought it was physiologically impossible. A funny thing happened the year after Roger Bannister broke the 4-minute mark, another runner beat his record less than 2 months later. Now thousands have broken the 4-minute barrier. Amazing huh?

The point is, you can get in shape, you can lose weight, and you can accomplish whatever you want in life. Within reason of course. One of my first job interviews I was asked by a panel of people what my primary goal was. I told them I wanted to be the first white guy on Soul Train. I later found out someone had already beat me to it. So pick out a goal that is ambitious, but still possible.

It is possible to totally change your life. No matter where you are now in life right now. I see it first hand in boot camp all the time. People that could barely walk for 5 minutes without being out of breath, now running 5Ks, 10Ks, and half marathons. These aren't professional athletes or actresses with every need taken care of; these are busy people just like you.

You know what the beauty of being really out of shape is? You can make MASSIVE progress by making simple changes in your life. You could start by lifting weights for 20 minutes twice a week, walking for 20 minutes a day twice a week, and practicing proper portion control. You would be amazed at what 80 minutes of exercise per week and a little mindful eating could do for you. Someone is changing their life right now, why aren't you?

There are a lot of people who are INTERESTED in losing weight and getting in shape, but are not COMMITTED. There is a huge difference in the two. When you are committed, nothing will stop you from reaching your goals. Not even pizza, birthday cake, alcohol, or weight loss plateaus will slow you down. When you are committed, every time you turn down those foods you feel stronger and it fuels your desire to succeed. When you are just interested, you feel deprived and cheated when you turn those foods down. It's the difference between being a conqueror and the conquered.

There are so many pitfalls out there that can trip you up. Try to drive more than 5 minutes without seeing a fast food place. If you aren't truly committed you will have trouble sticking to your goals. Want a great way to stay out of the fast food drive thru? Wrap your car with the phone number and web address of your fitness business. Maybe that just works for me... To stay committed you have to believe in the program you are doing, have someone to hold you accountable, and realize you are tougher than you think.

Don't skip around from exercise program to exercise program. Don't be on the South Beach Diet one week then the Atkins

Diet the next. You have to pick a lane and stick to it. Otherwise, how do you know what works and what doesn't? Seek out a program or trainer that you know works and put all of your effort into it. Do your research before beginning any exercise program or nutrition plan to make sure it is a good fit for you. If it is not something you can see yourself doing for the long run, why start? You have to believe that this is the program that will change your life. The key to getting where you want to be in life is consistency. In the past you have probably done great for a few weeks on your new fitness program and then fell off by the wayside. Just go look at the number of people in the gym in January compared to March for a real life example. Make the next one you start be the one that changes everything.

We all need to be held accountable. If people weren't held accountable for their actions, there is no way I would be throwing my money away on a mortgage every month. I would be buying pet kangaroos and teaching them to box with my money instead. Accountability can come in many different forms. It can be a trainer, a friend, or even as simple as a post on Facebook. People can stand to let their friends and family down, but not their adoring Facebook public! I gave up drinking coffee for Lent one time and put a post on Facebook saying I would pay anyone $100 that saw me drinking coffee. If you're cheap like me, that will work. You need that person that will push you in your workouts, that won't accept your excuses, and cares enough to tell you that failure is not an option. So ask yourself that tough question. Am I committed to reaching my goals or just interested?

I'm always amazed when I meet a mom who says she can't do something. Moms can do anything! When my son was born, I could not wait to get back to work. Don't get me wrong, I love my son more than anything in this world but the stay-at-home parent job is amazingly hard. Anyone that has been through pregnancy and childbirth can handle any exercise program out there. If guys were responsible for child birth, the human race would have died off years ago.

I often get asked why I do a boot camp for women only. There are several reasons why I do this. Women smell better, they are nicer, and are actually tougher than the men. We have done a few co-ed camps and the guys are absolutely exhausted within 20 minutes, while the women just keep plugging along. You can do more than you think, you are stronger than you think, and you are tougher than you think. Test yourself some time and you will see that I'm right.

Start developing your Fit Mom Mindset today. Every day is your chance to improve, so take advantage of it. Do you want to look back in 6 months and realize what you could have accomplished? Or do you want to look back and see how much you did accomplish? Whether you take 5 hours a week, 20 minutes a day or 5 minutes here and there, just do something for you!

You need it, you deserve it, and it is time to start working on the new you.

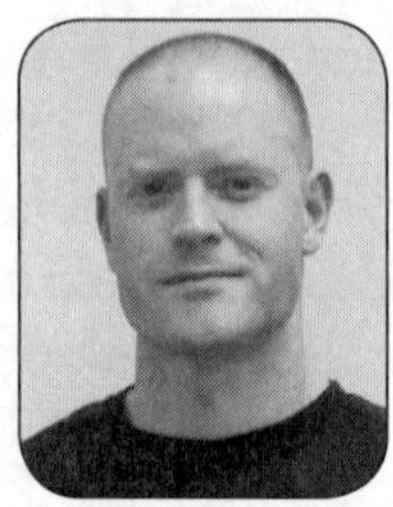

About Joe

Joe Martin is a NESTA Certified Adventure Boot Camp instructor, ACE certified personal fitness trainer, certified Sports Nutritionist, and certified Wellness Coach. He also holds a B.S. in Health Promotion with a Minor in Business from Auburn University.

Joe had been a lifelong athlete, until one day he woke up and realized he was 50 pounds overweight, depressed, and injured. It was a turning point in his life when he got fed up and realized there had to be a better way. From that day on, he has dedicated his life to studying health and fitness and using it to help others achieve their goals.

He has used this passion to train people from all walks of life, but specializes in fat loss for women. Known for his sense of humor and ability to make exercise fun, he has helped hundreds of people get their lives back through exercise.

To get your free copy of *30 Ways to Get Rock Solid Abs* visit:
www.HuntsvilleBootcamp.com to download it today.
You can also follow him on his blog at: www.JoeMartinFitness.com

CHAPTER 20

Balance – The Secret To Lasting Fitness

By Michael Coleman

When I turned 40, I weighed about 40 pounds more than I should. For years I have taught people how to keep in shape. Even so, I came to realize over time that updating my personal exercise and dietary protocols was needed to give me the health benefits I wanted. In this chapter I will show you how I adjusted my own training. Also, I'll explain how this journey of personal discovery taught me the three key principles which allowed me to reach my health and fitness goals in a short amount of time:

The **principle of MOVEMENT** helped me lose 45 pounds. Many of those pounds could easily be regained, however, so by following the **principle of LAUGHTER**, I discovered how to keep the weight off. I also realized how the **principle of GIVING** offered benefits that would consistently keep my body on track and my mind in a positive state.

I was anxious. My birthday was getting closer, and I began to worry about losing my edge. Watching those numbers on the scale go up, I began to reflect on my less-than-perfect eating habits. I knew that something had to be done!

To switch things up, I enlisted the help of a friend, a veteran United States Marine and personal trainer. He introduced me to a torturous training regimen consisting of traditional weights, machine, running and polymeric workouts. It didn't take long before I began to feel and see my body respond to the training: My muscles were definitely getting bigger, but I also began to notice some negative things:

- I got injured, including a very scary knee sprain.
- My belly wasn't getting any smaller.

Clearly I was over-training. My trainer's advice was factual but one-dimensional. I failed to see, at that time, that all three principles were necessary for balance. That in turn prevented me from noticing the warning signs.

MOVEMENT

I am a certified Yoga instructor and started studying the asanas (body postures) and pranayama

(breathing exercises) in 1986. It took me a while to learn, but one concept from that background really helped when I finally remembered to apply it to my wellness:

The basics are most important! A large percentage of some popular workouts are unnecessary at best and harmful at worst.

Without getting into too many complicated Sanskrit terms, most people interested in fitness have read the words *"Hatha Yoga"*. Hatha means sun & moon (like yin & yang in Chinese philosophy), and Yoga can be translated as the essence of union. The idea is to balance our bodies, and to bring our minds back into harmony.

My unbalanced training protocol was having the opposite effect, and I was developing repetitive-use injuries to prove it. While my trainer was out of town for several weeks, I decided to **decrease** the length of my solo workouts:

- I rested every other day.

- I consistently did eight basic yoga postures along with simple abdominal breathing.
- I reduced the amount of sets I did at the gym.
- I cut down on the minutes I spent on the treadmill, by sprinting and walking instead of long-distance running.

For 20 years, I've known that Hatha Yoga beginners are usually taught scores of poses. But I also have seen many students achieve **better** results from practicing only eight basic asanas (body postures). When I applied this concept to resistance training, I found that for a whole body workout I also only needed two sets of about eight basic exercises.

In a similar fashion, in my Yoga practice I stopped chasing after flashy contortions and concentrated on more simple and efficient techniques. In my experience, most people only need a slow, gentle practice of these eight basic postures:

1) A standing pose (like the forward fold)
2) A sitting pose (like sitting warrior or half lotus)
3) A backward-bending pose (like cobra or upward dog)
4) A forward-bending pose (like downward dog)
5) A leg-extension pose (like standing warrior I)
6) A twisting pose (like the lying spinal twist)
7) An inverted pose and counter pose (like shoulder stand, followed by fish)
8) A restorative pose (such as the 'corpse pose')

Something miraculous happened….I got STRONGER! When my trainer returned, we worked out together again. After the warm-up I stacked on the weight that I had been using for my Seated Pull-Downs. I finished the set easily and he said, "What have you been doing to get so strong?!" This scenario was repeated at other stations in the gym. Since I changed my philosophy, my injuries all healed and my joint pain has disappeared.

HOW I GOT RID OF MY BELLY

From my experience, I can certainly say that healthy nutrition – especially if fat loss is an issue – is just as much a product of how you eat as what you eat. Nutrition is a vast subject, so I'm focusing only on the time-tested basics. Also, after a little historical reference, I boiled down how I got rid of my extra belly fat into nine steps.

An ancient Yogic concept that food is *Sattvic* (calming, fresh, vegetarian & light), *Rajasic* (stimulating, spicy, etc., including some fish and poultry) or *Tamasic* (dulling, overcooked, heavy, including some red meat). There are two schools of thought in regards to this information: some say that in order to be healthy *all* of your food needs to be *Sattvic*, however others maintain that most foods can be consumed as long as your diet is balanced and toxic anti-nutrients are not eaten too excessively.

I have eaten all types of food in my life. I've found that certain kinds of food sit well with me and others absolutely do not. Also, I've noticed that what I eat now is radically different than what I enjoyed when I was a kid. – However, all that being said, I can tell you exactly what dietary considerations I followed to trim my waist quickly:

What to Eat

- I ate no foods containing high fructose corn syrup.
- I consumed only whole-grain or sprouted-grain bread. Also, I removed bread or crackers as "appetizers" at meals.
- I drank only water and tea (almost zero extra liquid calories).
- I switched to higher protein/lower calorie foods in my diet (e.g. choosing zero-fat Greek yogurt instead of regular, and wild Salmon rather than farm-raised).
- I ate raw, organic veggie salads regularly with no heavy dressings.

How to Eat

- I ate more frequently, and made sure I never missed breakfast. I also added a snack between lunch and dinner.
- Lunch was my largest meal.
- I ate no sweets after 5pm.
- I ate more slowly and was careful to enjoy my food.

If you do not already follow these or similar nutrition habits, you will certainly see positive results quickly by utilizing some or all of them.

LAUGHTER

After a recent emotionally-charged event in my personal life, I quickly gained 20 pounds! Up to that point, I would not have imagined just how much of an effect emotions could have on my health.

During that difficult period, I ate the same things and about the same calories as I normally did. Over-eating is not a big part of my coping mechanism. However, I still noticed that my posture, breathing, digestion, sleep patterns and other functions all changed for the worst, when I was feeling sad and lethargic, and vice versa. I know now from personal experience how much of a powerful difference negative thoughts can make on one's general health.

After I stopped feeling sorry for myself, I realized that I truly had the ability to change my state of mind by focusing on the more positive aspects of my situation. Whenever things got tough or I felt like stress was trying to derail me, I did two things that are both taught in Yoga:

- Straightened my posture
- Deepened my breathing

Those small but potent physical corrections gave me the opportunity to pause and reset. That time to reflect led to profound mental attitude adjustments that really helped me in daily life!

Your weight, like your life, will always have ups and downs. If we do not learn from these situations, I guess that we are doomed to repeat them. I survived a very difficult time in my life, regained a healthy body and got my vital energy back, because I did two things:

- Stopped having contempt for the education process and accepted "the waves of life" that I can't control.
- Focused on being constantly aware of how lucky (and thankful) I was to have the opportunities I did still possess.

RENT COMEDIES NOT DRAMAS

I found that the movies that I watched were part of my "mental nutrition." Until I was emotionally 100%, I felt that it was a good idea to starve my mind of any films that showcase too many problems without fun solutions (drama) or stress and fear producing action (horror). The bottom line to my successful mental diet, whether it's action, romantic or straight comedy, was to LAUGH more!

Laughter has been clinically proven to improve people's health. Even just smiling for 20 minutes a day has also been shown to have a noticeable effect on patients suffering from depression. Do your own research, and consider filling your movie queue with positive, mood-enhancing levity. I promise that your workouts will go faster, and your friends will enjoy your company more!

GIVING

In the beginning my fitness goals were pretty selfish and only about survival and ego. I think that most everybody starts from that place. Specifically:

- I wanted to have more functional longevity, by that I mean that I wanted to live a longer life AND also make sure that I still had enough mobility and energy to actual enjoy my golden years.

- I wanted to have a youthful body and a physique that would not make me feel ashamed at the beach.

What I Learned by Traveling the World

As a teacher, I was lucky enough to be able to see many of the most interesting and beautiful places in the world. From the thousands of people and hundreds of students that I've encountered, I realized that almost everybody shares similar problems and goals.

In an effort to identify some methods to help BOTH myself and others, these three problems: lack of *time*, lack of *information* and lack of *money* seem to be universal. As I found ways around these excuses for myself, I realized that only by *sharing* the answers could I really feel that my life had significance. Each country taught me an important lesson to share.

(i) Lack of Time

On the train to Germany, I passed through rustic vineyards, rolling countryside and the majestic Austrian Alps. By the time I reached Munich - exactly on time - it seemed that the whole world had changed....It was not just the Lederhosen and Dirndl dresses, but everywhere I looked there was an accurate clock, sometimes giant-sized.

Southern Germany has less of a reputation for being as stressed-out as the North, just go there during 'Oktober Fest' to see what I mean. But even at that time of the year, they find a way to get the job done. I've been acquainted with many engineers, including one at BMW headquarters. What I've gathered from their work-flow habits is simple but profound:

Consistently monitoring and adjusting the efficiency of our actions gives us the tools to produce maximum results with the minimum effort.

People with jobs frequently complain about not having enough time or energy to workout. Throughout this book, several time-saving strategies are discussed to make your workouts more efficient. Schedule your workouts each week and USE THEM! – You owe it to yourself.

(ii) Lack of Information

Shanghai, China, with a population of over 20 million people, is the very definition of "information over-load." In college, I studied some Chinese and later set out alone to deepen my cultural studies there.

Reading the language, many are daunted by the unfamiliar glyphs written in dark brushstrokes. But I was relieved and happy to learn that the thousands of traditional characters used in China all stem from only a few hundred word-pictures. Understanding that basic code is the key! It helps you to comprehend the more complicated ideas as just a combination of two or more related concepts. In essence, fitness is the same.

Like learning any foreign tongue, just slowly build your own "fitness language" that speaks to and resonates with you. Of course, new breakthroughs will continually be discovered. But, the *real* wisdom is in understanding the *process* of properly training yourself, and that will never change.

> *"Learn widely and go into what you have learned in detail so that in the end you can return to the essential."*
> ~ Mencius (an ancient Chinese philosopher)

(iii) Lack of Money

Overlooking the stunning beaches of *Ipanema* and *Copacabana*, the iconic *Christ the Redeemer* statue with its strong, stone arms outstretched stands guard over Rio de Janeiro, Brazil. Up close, I saw something that I had never noticed before. The 700 ton, soapstone monument has its heart *outside* its chest! I took this discovery as a curious sign.

In the shadow of the statue I met with some American university professors. That led to an invitation to visit a community center in the heart of *Cidade de Deus* (the City of God – an impoverished area outside of Rio that inspired a film of the same name).

It looked more like a prison yard than a fitness center. There were walls almost three meters high topped with razor-wire and guards wearing bullet-proof vests....Sponsored by a local factory, this was one of the only completely safe places for the children to play in their violent neighborhood.

Despite outward appearances, the children were sweet and their teachers were wonderful! I've traveled to many places in Brazil, so in my talk I was able to show examples and excite the kids about taking pride in just *being themselves*. They *could* find success with the resources they did have available.

Every country has low-cost fitness activities. Many of the most popular fitness "boot camps" are conducted in parks, on beaches or even on playgrounds. Personal trainers, gym memberships and special supplements can be expensive. ...But hospitals are even more expensive.

CONCLUSION

Each of us has the same job in life: to keep healthy and contribute as long as possible. Overcome lack of time, lack of information and lack of money excuses. Think of fitness training you do each week as an investment in your future and the future of your family.

Also, I've personally found that giving of your time, experiences and resources is the only path to lasting happiness and fulfillment!

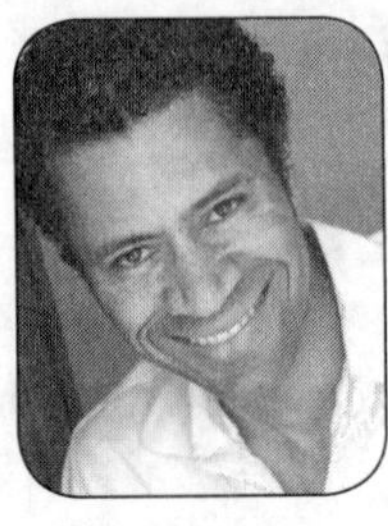

About Michael

Michael Coleman is a world-renowned expert of Asian movement, exercise and meditative arts. Starting his training in early childhood, Mr. Coleman is now one of the most highly regarded practitioners in the United States.

His wealth of teaching experience gives his readers an advantage in achieving their personal goals. He's traveled and taught extensively in Europe, South America and Asia, as well as conducted seminars in over 20 States in the US. For over two decades, Mr. Coleman has initiated thousands of people in the benefits of ancient health exercises - including yoga, breathing and vitality maintenance - in cities as diverse as Shanghai, Rio de Janeiro, and New York.

Mr. Coleman brings his unique experience to offer an "inner approach" to the otherwise external aspects of fitness training. He tirelessly promotes his mission of helping those in need in order to keep life in proper perspective. Michael has helped to raise tens of thousands of dollars in multiple projects benefiting the American and International Red Cross. In addition, some of Michael's clients and partners have been inspired to expand his work by helping in their local communities in numerous ways.

His numerous certifications, awards and acknowledgments include:

- Nationally Certified Yoga Instructor.
- Commendations for his teaching ability and community focus from the governor of his home state as well as from multiple city officials.
- Voted and named "Best of ...", "Editor's Choice" and one of four "Social Visionaries of 2010."
- Merited recognition from Brazil, Italy and other countries.

Learn more about Michael Coleman and how his life's work can help you. Go to: www.About.Me/Michael_Coleman for more information.

CHAPTER 21

Create Your Own Extreme Body/Life Makeover

By Kevin M. Harvey & Kristen Harvey DPT

KEVIN'S STORY

I was always picked on when I was a kid. I grew up and lived on a high school campus where my dad taught high school for 18 years. While growing up, my parents got me involved in a ton of extracurricular activities, like band, choir, and gymnastics, to keep me out of trouble. As a gymnast, I was a "skinny kid" and of course, was picked on a lot. That's probably the number one reason I started working out.

My role models were always bigger, stronger, and faster than me. They were also the most popular in school and the ones that got all the girls. In college, I started working out with weights in the basement of the guy's dorm. After my first workout, I was hooked. That summer, I gained a solid 30 pounds of pure muscle, going from a weak 165 lbs. to a lean, chiseled 195 lbs. Today, I stay between 210 lbs. and 215 lbs. Who's laughing now?!?

KRISTEN'S STORY

For as long as I can remember, I battled my weight.

I started exercising in 4th grade and counting calories at the age of 10.

I tried countless diets, owned a vast exercise video library, and had bookcases full of fitness books... But despite all the time, effort, and money I had invested, the more I tried to lose weight, the more I seemed to struggle.

It was my last year of graduate school when I hit my breaking point. I had become an out-of-control binge eater and with it, my self-confidence had plummeted, my depression was at an all-time high, and the girl in the mirror staring back at me was NOT the girl I knew or wanted to be.

One night, I was flipping through a fitness magazine when an article jumped off the page at me. It was about a woman who had completely transformed her body and life. Her before and after pictures were so astounding... I could NOT get it out of my mind! I wanted a story like hers. I wanted to model the same success she had had. So I hired her as my coach.

That decision became my turning point. In just 12 short weeks, I had lost 40 lbs. and dropped from a size 14 to a size 2. But more importantly, I regained control over my body and my eating habits again. My life was forever transformed.

The physical transformations Kevin and I experienced impacted us so deeply that it became our life's mission to help others experience the same things in their life. And for the past few years, we've been using many of those very same principles to help hundreds of men and women transform their lives and bodies like we did. I want to share with you the steps we took to help you achieve the same results in your life.

HOW TO CREATE YOUR OWN EXTREME BODY/LIFE MAKEOVER:

In order to make a change, we must first assess where we are starting.

Yes, I know… this is what everyone says. "Take your before pictures, your measurements, your starting weight…" yada, yada, yada… All this stuff is important. And I highly recommend it. But, if you don't dig deep from the very start, your fitness program or diet will only serve as a quick fix or temporary band-aid to a much bigger issue that will, once again, fail long-term when trying to achieve the body and life of your dreams. In order to create REAL dramatic, transformational change in your body and life, you must work diligently on the following three steps:

STEP #1 - CHANGE YOUR CURRENT BELIEFS.

It's been proven that we can never do anything consistently that is inconsistent with how we see ourselves. For example, you might have a goal to lose weight, but if you believe that you are fat and will always struggle with your weight, then there is a direct conflict between your goals and who you believe yourself to be. If there is a mismatch between your goals and your beliefs, your beliefs will always trump your goals. Why? Because unconsciously, we live and act according to our beliefs. Our life is a direct manifestation of how we see ourselves and what we believe. And if we only try to work on our goals at a conscious level, using tools like willpower, we'll struggle and eventually fall off track.

This sounds complicated, I know… There isn't a quick fix to change your beliefs and it won't happen overnight, but if you're willing to put in the time, it *will* happen and it will transform you from the inside out. This is your transformation game-changer. It's something I like to call "Effortless Transformation," where our unconscious mind automatically operates under new laws and principles which create new behaviors, habits, and ultimately, a new body and life. Because we're changing what we believe at a subconscious level, the changes that spring from it are effortless and automatic. The following 3 exercises will help you rewrite your beliefs and change the way you think…

a. **Become Aware of Your Current Conversation:** There is some type of debate going on in your head when you decide you're going to make a change. The first step in your transformation is becoming aware of what that conversation is and interrupting it if it isn't supporting your goals. So grab a pad of paper and a pencil and ask yourself the following questions:

- What are my goals and why are they important to me?
- What am I most frustrated with when it comes to achieving my goals?
- What have I tried in the past?
- Why haven't I achieved my goals?
- What excuses have I used before?
- What do I believe about eating healthy? Working out? Following a weight loss plan?

Write down what first comes to your mind. Don't be logical. Your beliefs aren't built that way... and when you convince yourself of something in a logical way, you're not getting a clear picture of how your brain really operates. Do these exercises FIRST before reading exercise two.

b. **Create a new vocabulary.** Look at your notes and notice what words you just used to describe your situation. Have you become aware of certain beliefs that are currently crippling your chances of success? Do you see a bunch of "I can't," "I won't," "I wish" or "If only's" on the page? These words shouldn't be allowed in your vocabulary. Become AWARE of the words you use and replace them with "I can," "I will" and "I choose to." Take your power back. You are in the driver's seat of your own life. Don't relinquish control to negativity and naysayers.

c. **Use Affirmations to Create New Beliefs.** In the first exercise, you became aware of beliefs you currently hold. Now it's time to throw out the beliefs that aren't supportive of your goals, and replace them with new beliefs. So ask yourself, "What beliefs do you need to have to help you reach your goals?" Once you know what they are, turn them into affirmations. Affirmations are declarations that state something to be true. Read these to yourself every day and say them with feeling! It might feel strange at first. But, if you commit to doing this every day for a couple weeks, your brain will start to replace old unsupportive beliefs with new beliefs that align with your goals.

From the very start of my transformation, my coach worked with me to help me change how I saw myself. During our initial consultation, I started to tell her my story. She immediately stopped me in my tracks and said, "Stop using a victim mentality! You are an athlete-in-training. I want you to think like an athlete, train like an athlete, and eat like an athlete." When she said that, a light came on in my brain. I had been playing victim and didn't even realize it. If I wanted to be successful, I had to start thinking like a champion. So my affirmation became, "I am an athlete. I think like an athlete, train like an athlete, eat like an athlete and look like an athlete." I repeated this to myself over and over again until I believed it. It gave me a sense of power, confidence, and excitement. And because I continually repeated this to myself, it soon became my identity. No longer did I believe I was a fat, lazy binge eater who would always struggle with her weight and never gain control. Creating this new belief was like adding rocket fuel to my goals: my new lifestyle became natural and enjoyable. As I began to eat like an athlete, train like an athlete and think like an athlete, I started to look like one, too.

So, to summarize step 1, you must first become aware of the beliefs that are holding you back. Then understand that you must replace them with new beliefs that align with and accelerate you towards your fitness goals. You do this by daily reciting powerful affirmations to yourself to rewire your brain and create new beliefs. Repetition is the mother of skill. You will become a different person only if you are willing to daily commit to feed your mind with positive thoughts and affirmations that install new beliefs and behaviors.

STEP 2 - ASSESS YOUR CURRENT SKILL SET AND DEVELOP THE SKILLS AND/OR ACQUIRE THE RESOURCES YOU NEED TO REACH YOUR GOALS...

Two of the biggest saboteurs of success are lack of confidence and lack of support. We can't do it all and we definitely don't know it all. A lack of confidence and support can often lead to fear of failure when trying to move forward. It's called "paralysis by analysis," and before we know it, we find ourselves "stuck" at a standstill.

a. **Identify where you might not be confident and fix it.** Do you have a goal but don't feel confident that you have the skill set needed to achieve that goal? If so, identify the areas where you aren't confident. You might know exactly what to do in terms of exercise but maybe you struggle with your diet and need some help. Do what you need to do to gain the confidence you require to achieve your goals.

   I personally believe everyone should have a coach or mentor. When you have a coach, you buy yourself speed through shortening the learning curve. Sure, you can do it on your own and experiment through trial and error, but you'll save yourself a lot of time and frustration by having someone else to guide you through.

b. **Build Your Dream Team.** The number one reason I see people fail is because of lack of support and accountability. Sometimes, when we are trying to make a change, we get a lot of resistance from those who are closest to us. It is at that point that you *must* step outside of your comfort zone and find new friends and accountability partners to help you in your fitness journey.

c. **Develop a Crystal Clear Vision for Your Transformation by Planning Your Results in Advance.** Know what you want and then focus on it with obsessive-like intensity until it becomes your reality. Your brain works in pictures and thrives on specificity. In other words, if you want to create a dramatic body transformation, you must PLAN YOUR RESULTS IN ADVANCE and create in your mind exactly what it is you want to achieve; the more details, the better.

If you aren't very clear on what you want to achieve, then take some time and thumb through some magazines or search the Internet, using sites like Google Images or Pinterest. Then create a vision board, whether it's a collage of pictures on a corkboard on your wall or a digital screensaver on your computer.

Once you've created your vision board, hang it up in your bedroom or someplace where you'll see it every day! Front of mind awareness is paramount. These pictures should be your source of inspiration DAILY as you move forward towards your goals. It'll help you create laser-like focus on achieving your dreams. The late Jim Rohn used to say, "Obstacles are what you see when you take your eyes off your goals," so make sure that you stay FOCUSED on your goals and use the VISION board to help you zero in with extreme CLARITY on what you're trying to achieve.

STEP #3 - PLAN YOUR WORK AND WORK YOUR PLAN.

Most people have two identities: a shell identity and a core identity. The shell identity is where you currently are if you're reading this. It's the place you probably didn't plan to be and definitely not where you wanted to be.

The core identity is your true identity or who you really want to be. If there was no limit to what you could achieve and who you could be, this would be the way you'd be living your life; your dream body, your ideal lifestyle, and your life without limits. The real key to shed your shell and uncover your core identity is that you need to take the actions and do what is consistent with that identity.

a. **"Don't talk about it. Be about it!"** Planning is important but all the planning in the world is no match to those who take action. Remember, actions become habits through repetition. Therefore, if you want to bridge the gap between who you are and who you want to be, you must take the actions consistent with your goals. The more you do it, the more natural it will become.

b. **Commit to Kaizen.** (The Japanese term for "continuous improvement.") If you've achieved your goals and you're reaching new heights, CONGRATULATIONS! But it's not the end! It's only the beginning.

We often set a goal and work really hard to achieve it. Then, when the competition ends or whatever it may be, we're left wondering "Now what?" It takes from a couple weeks to months to rewire our brain and create new patterns and new ways of thinking. But it takes only a few days to undo it. In order to fully experience life and reach your true potential, you must continually push your boundaries and challenge yourself. So *commit to kaizen* and you will achieve a life beyond your wildest dreams!

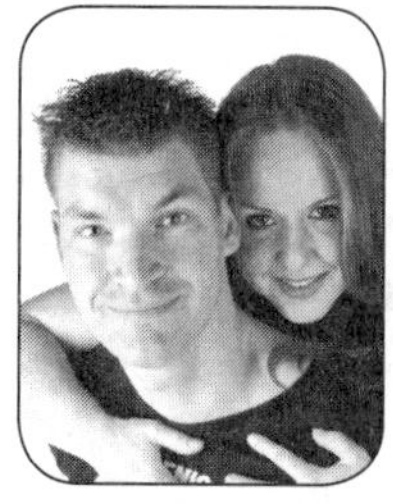

About Kevin & Kristen

Both Kevin and Dr. Kristen Harvey's passion for fitness started at a very early age, but it wasn't until they transformed their bodies that they knew it would become their life's mission. And for the last several years, the Harveys have been helping elevate and empower ordinary people to live powerful, passionate and purpose-driven lives through their company, Scenic City Adventure Boot Camp, in Chattanooga, TN. With over 20 years combined experience in the fitness industry, the Harveys are passionate about finding new, exciting ways to make food and fitness fun, so that everyone will CRAVE a healthy lifestyle.

Blush magazine calls this fitness duo the "unstoppable husband-and-wife team." Since 2007, their signature boot camps and body transformation contests have helped 1000's of people change their bodies faster and easier than ever. In 2011, they were voted #1 in personal training by the *Chattanooga Times Free Press* "Best of the Best" contest. The Harveys have appeared on ABC, CBS, NBC, FOX, several local radio stations and in print interviews. They have consulted for companies such as Sherwin Williams, the University of TN, and the TN Dept of Education, and are monthly fitness columnists for *Family News Network* magazine.

Kevin received his Bachelor's degree in Corporate/Community Wellness Management with a minor in Business and Physical Education. He holds several national fitness certifications ranging from group exercise to personal training, with an understanding of nutrition and psychology.

Dr. Kristen Harvey received her Doctor of Physical Therapy from the University of Tennessee at Chattanooga in 2007. She holds several certifications in personal training, sports nutrition, healthy cooking, and functional movement.

Kristen's 2020 vision is to help elevate and empower 1,000,000 overweight women to take back control of their life and transform their bodies from the inside out, using the effortless transformation principles. She recently launched Help Me Lose Weight TV, to cultivate a community of like-minded women who are ready to transform their bodies and live a life without limits. You can get a Free Copy of her 7-day *"Make Me Over*" meal plan and

"Calorie-Crushing Workout" tear-out sheet by visiting: http://www.helpmeloseweight.tv.

To learn more about Scenic City Boot Camp's nutrition programs and fitness services and how you can try them out for 2 weeks risk-free, please visit: http://www.ScenicCityBootCamp.com.

CHAPTER 22

Unlocking the Code

By Gregg Viscuso

Wellness is not the lack of poor health; it is a series of lifestyle choices that support good health and well being. It is giving the body what it needs to create optimal health.

Wellness and the pursuit of wellness are all over the news and internet. There are many opinions on why the topic is on everyone's mind. The first is the new healthcare reform act has been signed by the US government. Secondly, health insurance companies and employers wanted to lower their skyrocketing health care cost. Baby boomers are getting older and they are searching for ways to stay healthy and be more productive. Whatever the reasons are, everyone is searching for answers on how to achieve wellness.

So why are we searching for these answers? Weren't we all told since we were children to eat a "low-fat" diet and go out for a walk or jog and all would be fine? Let's examine how that worked out for all of us. The Centers for Disease Control and Prevention 2010 report states the following:

- About one-third of U.S. adults (33.8%) are obese.
- Approximately 17% (or 12.5 million) of children and adolescents aged 2—19 years are obese.

- During the past 20 years, there has been a dramatic increase in obesity in the United States and rates remain high. In 2010, no state had a prevalence of obesity less than 20%. Thirty-six states had a prevalence of 25% or more.

The graph below comes from the National Health and Nutrition Examination Survey (NHANES), the Behavioral Risk Factor Surveillance System (BRFSS), and the U.S. Department of Agriculture (USDA).

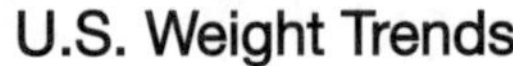

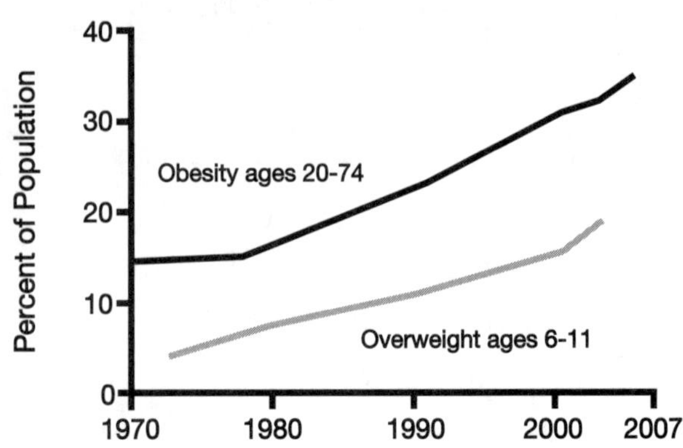

What happened? How could we have all of this information and be the unhealthiest, most overweight generation of all time? We have so much information from magazines, internet, and infomercials. We hear: drink coffee it is healthy, no don't drink coffee it is unhealthy, same with eggs and milk and gluten!! How do we sort it all out? Sometimes I feel as if my head will explode with all of the conflicting information.

This was the dilemma I was in years ago. My passion in life is to keep as young, active and healthy as possible. I want to look good, feel good, have energy and enjoy my children, their children and possibly their children! When I say enjoying them, I mean running around and playing with them, not sitting in a rocking chair watching them.

So I set out on a mission to unlock the wellness code! My objectives were clear. Gather the most trustworthy information on wellness as I could, and spread the word to everyone that had the same goals as I.

Here is my journey….

I was born in 1963 of Italian and Czechoslovakian heritage. I unfortunately did not receive "gifted genetics." I graduated high school at 5' 11" and a paltry 128 lbs. You can only imagine the jokes that were made…. "Hey is that a string hanging from your shirt? Oh no, it is your arm!" Very funny I know.

During my life's journey, I have found that unfortunate circumstances seem to be a wonderful motivator and growth opportunity if you focus on the positive of a situation instead of the bad. So with this philosophy in place, I was on my way. I started to work out and eat as healthy as I could. My goal was simply and straight forward: Gain weight, gain respect and to be brutally honest, gain my first date.

Jump forward one year and the transformation has begun. My weight jumps to 175 lbs., my bench press and squat nearly double, and true success, my first girlfriend! Everything seemed to be going well but something un-expectantly happened, my confidence start to soar, my grades in college improved, I start to take leadership roles, my energy levels rose and my physician told me that my cholesterol has dropped by 60 points. All of this occurs while all I wanted was to look better! That is when I was hooked, I had searched for one goal but what I unexpectedly received was the gift of wellness.

Flash forward five years and my passion for fitness has led me into the pharmaceutical world. How better to promote well-being than teaching physicians about life-changing medicines. This, coupled with training clients on wellness, and I was set to accomplish my second goal of spreading the health and wellness word.

During my early years as a pharmaceutical representative, I visited one of the top physician's offices to promote my medicine.

As I arrived there I saw a line of six other Pharmaceutical Representatives with the same goal as myself, to convince the doctor to use their medicine instead of a competitor's. While in the waiting room, as this unfolds, I ask myself the question; How will this physician sort out all of the information he/she is about to receive? Who does he/she believe, what information will they trust and why? The decisions they make can be ones of life and death. I thought this is the same position I and so many others have when trying to uncover the correct information towards wellness, nutrition and fitness.

That is when it hit me! BAM!! If I could discover the process physicians go through deciding what medicine a patient should receive, then I can incorporate the same process towards wellness. I could now give advice with the same confidence that physicians have when making one of the most important decisions about health.

I started my discussion as usual with the physician. After I finished, I asked the question, "How do you sort through all of the information and determine what is most effective and safest for your patients?" He replied, "Gregg, that is a great question that every physician must resolve." That is why the medical profession has developed a method called "Evidence-Based Medicine."

This is what led me to unlocking the Wellness Code. Let me first explain "Evidence-Based Medicine."

Wikipedia describes that **Evidence-based medicine (EBM)** aims to apply the best available evidence gained from the scientific method to clinical decision-making.[1] It seeks to assess the strength of evidence of the risks and benefits of treatments (including lack of treatment) and diagnostic tests.[2] Evidence quality can range from meta-analyses and systematic reviews of double-blind, placebo-controlled clinical trials at the top end, down to conventional wisdom at the bottom.

What does that really mean? Let me explain. One of the most

important decisions a physician has to make is what therapy they need to put a patient on to make their health outcome improve the best – what is not only a good medicine, but what is **BEST** with the least amount of side effects. Let's look at an example of EBM.

A patient goes to the doctor's office because they have been having frequent stomach pain. After a full evaluation to rule out any other underlying problems the doctor has determined that they have GERD (Gastro Esophagus Reflux Disease) or "heartburn." The physician now implements EBM to determine the most effective course of therapy. With the background of reading medical journals and numerous studies on this topic, the doctor can now determine what to prescribe.

Years ago, the doctor would prescribe any medicine that worked better than simply doing nothing. Now, as time has passed, there are many new treatments to choose from, and there are many more scientific studies comparing these new treatments. EBM was developed to answer the following question: What is not only an effective treatment, but what is the **MOST** effective treatment?

To answer this, they turn to the most prestigious peer-reviewed Medical Journals that publish studies that compare two different treatments in head-to-head trials. These trials have strict guidelines on how to determine the best therapy. After the studies are completed, each Medical Journal then reviews the methods and results of the trial to determine if it is a credible study.

After reviewing the studies and knowing what studies are more credible than others, the physician determines that the best way to treat this patient is to use a PPI (Proton Pump Inhibitor). They could have used an antacid or an H2 blocker, but EBM clearly shows that PPIs work better.

Now we know how physicians go about making their decisions using EBM. We must also note that they only use studies that are the most reliable. In medicine and even more in wellness, there are some poor studies that are designed and the researchers try to influence the outcome of the study. We just can't believe any study, we must look at the studies that are designed to prevent any biases.

There are many ways to design a study. Physicians and scientists have created a list of the most reliable study designs down to the least reliable. Here is a list of designs with the first being the most trusted:

1. Randomized-controlled trials; Controlled trials (non-randomized)
2. Cohort Studies; Case-Controlled Studies; Well-designed retrospective studies
3. Meta-analysis; Expert opinion/clinical guidelines
4. Case reports, animal and in-vitro studies

Let's now look at wellness and see how we can utilize this method to help us unlock the wellness code. This is where I discovered the most important news in wellness, **EBFN (Evidence-Based Fitness and Nutrition)**. When utilizing EBFN we examine the scientific studies, determine which are credible, and then we compare each method to determine the **MOST** effective form of fitness and nutrition. It is important to recognize credible scientific studies and how to analyze the results.

This process takes years to accomplish. It is also incredibly expensive since you must subscribe to all of the top journals around the world. Fortunately, there are people out there that do all of the work for you.

Let's now look into fitness and nutrition to review two examples of using bad scientific information to make important choices.

Everyone is on a mission to lose weight. When this is their goal, they focus on one area "cardio." You see them on the first nice day in the spring going out for a jog or they will be in every gym in America on the bike, treadmill or the stepper! Why? Is aerobics the *best* way to lose weight?

Remember the above story with the patient who had stomach pains? The physician didn't choose a medicine that worked better than doing nothing, they choose the *best* medicine. Can cardio help you lose weight? Maybe, but it takes hours and hours and the results are minimal at best. When we look at EBNF, the science tells us that a **four minute workout can burn 900% more fat than 45 minutes of long, boring aerobics!!** If we are all too busy to work out, why would anyone go out for a jog when we could work out for four minutes and increase our results nine-fold?

Let's look at the second example. Let's tackle the message we have all heard from the government, our physicians and everything we read as we grew up. "Eat a low fat diet, high in carbohydrates, and you will lose weight, decrease your risk of heart attacks and diabetes and improve your overall health.

Did you ever wonder where the "low fat" craze began? How about the science behind it? It must have been overwhelming since the NIH, Food and Nutrition Board of the National Academy of Science, the government's Food Guide Pyramid and the American Medical Association all agreed it was the way to control our health.

Until the late '70's, the accepted wisdom was that fat and protein protected against overeating by making you satisfied and that carbohydrates made you fat.

Enter Ancel Keys, a University of Minnesota physician who introduced the low-fat-is-good-health dogma in the 50's. He proposed that dietary fat raises cholesterol levels. Since higher cholesterol levels were associated with higher heart attack rates, then eating less fat would decrease heart attacks.

This is called a "leap of faith" in science! Unfortunately, it's an imperfect world. Ancel was trying to associate an increase of dietary fat to an increased body fat. There was only one big problem, there were absolutely NO studies to confirm this.

When using this "leap of faith" philosophy in January of 1977, a Senate committee led by George McGovern published its "Dietary Goals for the United States," advising that Americans significantly curb their fat intake to abate an epidemic of "killer diseases" sweeping our country. In 1984 the National Institute of Health officially recommended eating less fat of *any* kind.

Bam! a new industry was born, "low–fat" everything! Low fat milk, yogurt, cheese, cookies, and chips, you name it and we were taking the fat out of it and we had to replace it with something that still made it taste yummy so we added sugar and or high fructose corn syrup.

The result of "bad science" or in this case NO science, we currently eat an extra 400 calories a day, increase our grain consumption by 60 pounds, and our sugar (high fructose corn syrup) by 30 additional pounds. That has lead us for the first time seeing Type 2 diabetes in children, the highest levels of adult diabetes, and the obesity epidemic we now experience. All in the word of "bad" science!

As we have seen by the two above examples, deciding who and what to believe can be somewhat overwhelming in the world of wellness. It would be nearly impossible for anyone to research all of the data and sort out what is credible and what is junk. That is why it is so important to receive information from a trusted source that knows how to find, uncover and interpret the latest scientific data in an Evidence-Based Nutrition and Fitness way.

When you utilize EBFN you receive fitness and nutrition information that is proven to get the best results in the least amount of time. No more will you have to read the small print or look at unproven before-and-after pictures that just can't be believed. How nice would it be to know that the information you received is not only effective but it is MORE effective than any other method? …always knowing you will have the most trustworthy information available – saving thousands of dollars on worthless products, supplements and false claims!

The answer is out there, you just have to go out and seek it. I promise you one thing for sure – you will know it when you find it. All of your goals of looking great, feeling great, increased energy, healthy sex life, and a positive mental attitude all can be yours in much less time than you ever thought possible. It is wonderful to wake up every day and feel as good as you did in your prime no matter what age you are. The greatest gift in the world I have received is informing as many people as I can on the wonders of wellness!

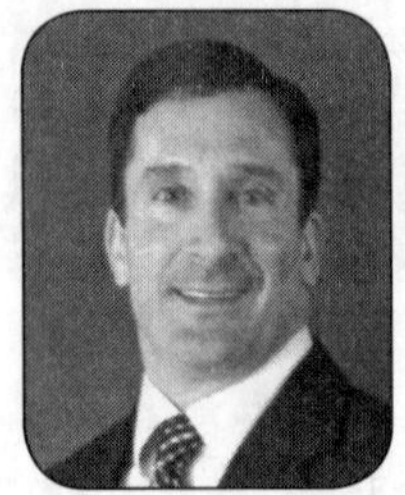

About Gregg

Gregg Viscuso, President, wellnessiD; Corporate Wellness Trainer; Certified in Exercise and Sports Nutrition; Body Transformation Specialist.

Gregg is a former wimpy kid and a self-proclaimed "work in progress" that has tried and perfected many methods of exercise over the years. After 27 years of using trial and error, and the power of Evidence Based Fitness and Nutrition (the practice of using scientific studies to compare different exercise and diet protocols to determine which is the most effective), he now is ready to share all of his years of work and study to get you in the healthiest shape of your life!.

Upon graduating from college he has worked in the Pharmaceutical Industry for 25 years. He has seen firsthand that physicians need a "go to" source they can count on with scientific knowledge, the ability to teach, and a passionate person who wants everyone to enjoy each day of their life with health, vim and vigor!!! They value and trust his opinions! As a former high school athlete and a life-long workout junkie, he discovered his calling was to empower others to forever change their bodies and lives for the better. Gregg has the unique ability to translate his own personal failures into remarkable successes for the people he works with.

Gregg is best known as the owner of wellnessiD LLC, http://www.wellnessid.net where physician's patients, corporations, and everyday people go to find the Holy Grail of Wellness. By using Evidence-Based Fitness and Nutrition, Gregg answers the ultimate question; What is the fastest and most effective way to work out and eat to be the healthiest and fit I can be? If you would like to know more about the answer, please visit: www.wellnessid.net

Gregg is also widely considered to be the area's leading fitness boot camp expert. He owned and operated *West Chester Fit Body Boot Camp* in West Chester, PA, which featured 30-minute express metabolic boot camp workouts for busy professionals looking to optimize body composition, performance, and overall health.

Gregg is also a Corporate Fitness and Health Trainer for one of the largest Pharmaceutical companies in the world. Here he works with all level of employees to increase their everyday energy, improve their nutrition and help them with goal setting and stress reduction. With the rising health costs, employers have discovered that an active and healthy lifestyle benefits the company as employees have more energy, less sick days and a more positive attitude that all benefit the bottom line!!! He conducts live presentations for corporations on fitness, nutrition and stress reduction. He can even bring his world-renowned boot camps directly to your work place.

Gregg is also passionate about helping fitness professionals all over the world by helping more people in order to solve the raging obesity epidemic crippling our world. He lectures as a presenter for his expertise in fitness and nutrition program design and his knowledge in Sports and Exercise Nutrition, in which he is certified.

Gregg also trains young athletes at all level to become stronger, increase speed and agility, and enhance their nutrition. Many of his athletes have achieved scholarships at Division 1 and Division 2 colleges. Gregg has also had the pleasure to watch some of his athletes make it to the professional sports level! Not only have athletes achieved their goals by using his workouts and nutrition advice, but everyday people have also reached their goals as his programs have been used nationally.

To learn more about Gregg Viscuso and wellnessiD, please visit:
http://www.wellnessid.net and his
email address is: wellnessid@gmail.com

In Health and Wellness!

CHAPTER 23

Change Your Lifestyle, Change Your Life

10 Simple Steps to a Happy, Healthy You!

By Justine SanFilippo

You look in the mirror one day and don't recognize yourself. Your pants are tight, you have bags under your eyes, and oh my goodness, is that a gray eyebrow hair? You feel haggard, stressed, tired, and rely on caffeine to get you through the day. That late-night glass of wine has become a necessity to unwind rather than a luxury. To top it off, a full night's sleep is something you read about once in a fairy tale....

What happened to get you to this point? Life happened. Other things became a priority and you are at the bottom of the list. The kids, wife, husband, dog, job and house are #1 and you are last.

I remember the day I didn't recognize my reflection in the mirror. Life had taken various pieces of me and all that was left was a teeny, tiny speck.

When I was 15, I got bit by the "modeling bug." This began when I was asked to attend modeling school. Soon after I got a couple modeling jobs, decided to enter a beauty pageant, and fell in love with the industry. I wanted to be a model.

My love for the modeling industry continued after graduating from the University of Notre Dame. By then I realized I'd rather work behind the scenes to learn more about the industry. I found a job as an intern for an agency in New York City. My ultimate goal was to be a Booker for a well-known agency. Eventually I was promoted to Assistant, then finally to my "dream job" as a Booker! I was excited, but nervous too. Could I keep up the pace? By this point, I had no life, no time to take care of myself, no sleep, poor eating habits, and was just plain exhausted. But I was happy, right?

A short time after reaching this goal, my dream came to a screeching halt. One morning, exhausted as usual, I answered the phone to a client. The client called back and complained about my phone etiquette. Apparently, sleep-talking was not acceptable, and they were right. My boss took me aside and I realized I just couldn't do it anymore. If you've seen the movie *"The Devil Wears Prada,"* the depiction isn't far from the truth. Keep up with the pace or get out of the way!

In hindsight, if I had followed the 10 Simple Steps I'm about to show you, I would have kept more balance in my life. I achieved my "dream job," but the other areas of my life fell by the wayside. The modeling bug had died. What looked back at me in the mirror was a stranger I barely recognized. Now what?

I had to re-evaluate my life, my goals, face my fears and move forward into unknown territory. Through self-assessment and realizing what my true passion is, I now have a *new* dream – to be happy and healthy and help others do the same. I'm going to share with you what I learned in *10 Simple Steps* so you can achieve wellness and balance in your OWN life and be proud of what you see in the mirror every day!

STEP 1 – HONESTY IS THE BEST POLICY

This first step may be the hardest, but it is the most important. You have to be honest with yourself. Answer this question – *ARE YOU HAPPY?*

Now, your immediate gut reaction is the correct answer. With each passing moment, you may be inclined to change your initial answer to some compromise. As you think about it, you may say "I'm happy most days" or "I'm happy in some parts of my life" or "I feel guilty saying no because I feel I should say yes."

After answering this seemingly simple, yet loaded question, now you have a starting point.

Take three steps back and look at your life objectively. This is probably the second hardest thing to do (we're getting the tough ones out of the way first!). When examining your life, which areas need to be changed? There's always room for improvement. Areas that may need attention are: Diet, Physical Activity, Career, Relationships, Stress, Sleep, Relaxation, Fun, Finances, Home Environment, Social Life, and Health. Broad categories, I know, but they're all tied together. As you work on one area, the others will automatically be altered in a domino effect. So, don't stress yourself out and think you have to work on ALL these areas all at the same time. Stress leads to excess cortisol, which leads to excess belly fat, which leads to more cortisol, and the merry-go-round continues.... I'll make this process simple – let's narrow down which areas need the most attention. Time to make a list!

STEP 2 – MAKE A LIST AND CHECK IT TWICE

I'm sure even Santa has his work/life balance issues, especially around the holidays, so let's follow his lead and start with a list. This list will consist of the 5 most important areas of your life that you would like to change. Feel free to choose from the areas listed in Step 1. For example, you may choose:

1. Lose weight
2. Reduce stress
3. Spend more time with family
4. I hate my job and need a new one
5. Have more fun

Now that you have your list, it's time to check it twice.... and prioritize.

STEP 3 – PRIORITIZING FOR "DUMMIES"

You are not a dummy. In fact, you are extremely smart for reading this book! Many of us, however, are "dummies" when it comes to our priorities. We have them completely backwards, upside-down and sideways. Everybody and everything else comes first and we are last. Let's set our priority of which area to focus on.

When you look at your list above, each area may initially seem equally important. The simplest way to prioritize is to answer one question – Which area affects ALL the other areas the most? For example, when I had my "dream job," I had no time for myself, so I felt like crap. I felt like crap, so I ate crappy food. I ate crappy food, so I had no energy. I had no energy, so I had nothing left to give to anyone or anything. In this domino effect, "career" was the biggest culprit affecting every area of my life. Take a moment and renumber your list. Whichever area affects the others the most is what should be tackled first!

Now let's get over your fear of change…

STEP 4 – FEAR IS YOUR NEW BFF

Someone once told me that when you feel fear, you are exactly where you need to be. If you are about to do something, go somewhere, or experience something new and you feel butterflies, you are in the right place. You are about to grow and change… for the better!

I learned from a favorite book of mine it is common to experience fear, but to do what you fear the most anyway. Feel the fear, embrace it, and do it anyway. Only by facing our fears do we grow. We are never given something we can't handle, so keep that in mind next time you feel butterflies in your tummy.

In general, people don't like change. We like comfort, familiarity, and routine. There is some benefit to that, but after a while you become stagnant. Changing any part of our life can be scary because what happens next?

What if I *do* lose the weight? Will my friends hate me and be jealous? What if I *do* find a new job? Will my current coworkers write me off? What if I *do* tell my significant other what I've been feeling? Will he or she reject me? The list could go on and on. The bottom line is, what we fear the most is FEAR OF FAILURE.

Wow, that's a 'doozy!'

Let's retrain our brain to define what failure *truly* is. Failure is NOT EVEN TRYING. *So what* if you lose the weight and your "friends" become jealous of you? You'll meet new people with your newfound confidence and make new friends. *So what* if you get a new job and your current co-workers don't talk to you again? You'll meet other great co-workers at your new job. *So what* if your significant other doesn't respect your feelings once you share them? It's probably a sign you should go start fishing for someone else. The answer to any fear is.... SO WHAT!!

If you change your perception of failure, it's really not that scary. Failure is not even trying. Once you're past the idea that there really is no failure, there really is no fear. That's why fear is your new BFF. She's really a friend in disguise.

STEP 5 – MANY SMALL STEPS FOR YOU = ONE GIANT LEAP FOR YOUR LIFE

You're ready for change, you've made a list of areas to focus on, you've defined the most important area, and you're over your fear. Now it's time to break it down into realistic baby steps!

I'm a big fan of baby steps. One thing many people do is set too high a goal in an unrealistic timeframe. When they don't achieve it, they give up. If a person wants to lose 20 pounds in a day, that's not realistic. They're setting themselves up for disappointment. The better way would be to learn about the healthy ways to lose weight and keep it off, and then set small goals around their findings.

It's time to educate yourself on which steps are needed to reach your end goal. If you want a new job, what do you need to do? You can't **poof** have a new job tomorrow that will meet all of your expectations. Of course, if you had a genie in your pocket doling out wishes, it would be easy.

Since your genie is currently busy, write down 10 small steps that are needed to achieve your goal. For example, with finding a job, the first 3 steps might be:

1. Update resume
2. Research companies
3. Apply for one job a day, etc.

Whether it's losing weight, finding a job, restructuring your finances, preparing for retirement, or reducing stress, each major change involves many teeny, tiny steps.

Look at your list of baby steps and write next to them a realistic time frame you feel to accomplish each one. Some will be a few days, others a few weeks and others a few months or so. BE REALISTIC. Then keep yourself accountable. Put your actionable baby steps in plain sight – on your phone, on your calendar, or on your bathroom mirror. If you need extra accountability, ask a friend to help!

Baby steps are a way to witness your progress. It is VERY rewarding to cross something off the list! You've accomplished something and are moving in the right direction. All of these steps add together to one giant leap. Now it's time to move those legs.

STEP 6 – READY, SET, ACTION!

I still love the entertainment industry and always will, so for the moment we'll pretend I'm your Assistant Director. You are the Director and in charge of your life. It's time to roll the camera and take action!

You're going to direct your own movie – your life – and you can't do it sitting on the couch in pajamas. Scene One. Take One. Ready. Action....

As you accomplish each baby step, reward yourself. Go out to lunch, go to a movie, get a massage – whatever makes you happy. Rejoice in the success! So you got to Step 8 and not Step 9 yet. Is that failure? No. The eight things you accomplished are moving you forward! There is no failure because you are taking action, so pat yourself on the back. Be proud of yourself and continue on your path. The world is waiting to see your directorial debut!

STEP 7 – PAY ATTENTION TO YOUR SURROUNDINGS

As you continue to take small steps, rejoice in your accomplishments and get closer to your overall goal, why is it some people seem to sabotage your efforts? You're on a diet, and your boyfriend brings home pizza. You're excited about pursuing your lifelong dream as an artist, but your "friends" say it's not a real career.

Sometimes people, inadvertently or on purpose, may try to derail you.

Look at those around you and rate how they generally make you *feel* on a scale of 1-10. 1's are folks that drag you down and make you feel bad about yourself, and 10's are those that uplift, support, and empower you. The 1's will bring you down to their level (think gravity). It's much easier to sink downwards than go against gravity and move upwards.

As you pursue your goals, pay attention to your surroundings. If anyone is dragging you down, literally, it's time to cut the cord. Only hang around those that uplift you. Antigravity is cool.

STEP 8 – MAKE FRIENDS WITH CHALLENGES .... AND KEEP MOVING FORWARD!

Fear is your new BFF, and Challenges are her siblings! As you go along your journey, you will run into obstacles and unpaved roads. How to face challenges? Bring it on! You have to go down several roads to find the best route to your destination. With each roadblock comes an opportunity to grow.

You went on a job interview you really wanted and didn't get it. So what! There is a job that's a *better* fit waiting out there for you. Don't stop the process of seeking different roads when you hit an obstacle. Because of your actions to move forward, the job that's the best fit for you *will happen.*

And as long as you are *moving* in the direction towards your goal, the right people, places, and opportunities will open up to you. You just have to keep *moving.*

STEP 9 – YOU DON'T HAVE TO BE PERFECT

Perfection is unrealistic. We want to be the perfect mom or the perfect dad or the perfect employee. If I learned anything from the modeling industry, it's that nobody's perfect. How boring would it be if we were all perfect? If we were all the best at everything, the best looking, the smartest, and were the most successful? Completely boring. Everyone is perfect in their imperfection, and that's what makes you interesting and unique. So, remove the pressure of trying to be perfect – it's exhausting. Accept who you are and be the best you can be for yourself.

STEP 10 – MIRROR, MIRROR ON THE WALL.... I SEE MYSELF... AND I AM HAPPY!

After all is said and done, the ultimate goal is to be happy and proud of yourself. To look in the mirror and love what you see. You look rested, your pants are looser, and that darn gray eyebrow hair is still there. But, with a touch of gray comes wisdom. You've accomplished something, so be proud of yourself! You have taken small steps to ultimately change your life. You are learning to love yourself and take care of the person you are, inside and out.

The domino effect of the steps you have taken will begin to unfold - all that was needed was a little push. Happiness is now yours for the taking – because you *deserve* to be Happy and Healthy!

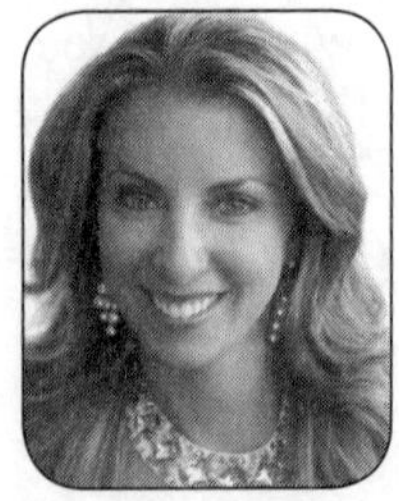

About Justine

Justine SanFilippo graduated from the University of Notre Dame with a Bachelor's degree in Business Administration. Since college, she found her passion in health, wellness and nutrition! She attended the Institute for Integrative Nutrition® in New York City in 2005 and became a Certified Health Coach - www.happyhealthyweightloss.com. She is also an ACE Certified Personal Trainer and enjoys training others to help them reach their fitness goals. She is currently pursuing her Masters in Human Nutrition with plans to pursue her PhD. She writes a weekly blog filled with practical nutrition and wellness tips at: www.happyhealthypeople.com and she also sends out a free monthly newsletter.

Justine loves to teach others about health, wellness and nutrition, and she enjoys helping others achieve their weight-loss goals. Prior to relocating to Austin, TX, she was the owner a women's gym in New Jersey where she spread the message of health and wellness to the members.

Justine has several books in the works. The first will be a book called *"Lose Your Inches Without Losing Your Mind!"©* Afterwards, she will come out with her children's book series.

"Lose Your Inches Without Losing Your Mind!"© is an honest and realistic approach to losing inches in a healthy, balanced way.... and keeping them off! She uses her past experience with diets (and losing 45 lbs!) to relate to others how to finally reach their ideal size. It is a fun and quick read – no dieting allowed in this book!

Her children's book series will teach the children (and their parents!) about making healthy choices in an easy and memorable way, especially when they are young and most impressionable. There are many instances of child obesity that she feels can be altered positively. Educating both children and their parents in a simple, easy-to-understand way is how she hopes to make a difference.

She looks forward to continuing to educate as many people as possible through her books, articles, seminars and speaking engagements. Her ultimate goal is to help individuals of all ages, sizes, and walks of life be HAPPY, HEALTHY PEOPLE!

CHAPTER 24

Flex Your Joy

By Dorothy Jantzen

What is Joy?

Joy is the feeling of great delight or happiness. The state of joy is what many call our natural state – the state of true happiness where all resistance has fallen away.

When we experience "Joy" we can connect with our inner-knowing, Spirit or God and be our best selves. We "lighten up." We're released from stress, fear, and other negative emotions allowing us to be more open, kind, loving and generous. The cells of our body get a break from constant stress and do what they are meant to do… thrive, rebuild, and heal!

I use the term "*Flex* your Joy" to mean exercise body and mind to connect to Joy.

Obviously, this is easier said than done.

Our modern lifestyle does not promote living in Joy, rather, it perpetuates stress. We are told we *deserve* to have fun, and that the *journey* is the reward, however, this is incongruent with the demands of society. Whether tending to families or jobs, we constantly face pressure and deadlines to do more, and we multitask at every opportunity. Day after day, we get up and do, do, do and then do, do some more. *And yet we don't seem to be getting anywhere!*

The result is we take less and less time to care for ourselves, our bodies and to connect to our Joy. We too often feel lethargic, sad or cranky. We know we could treat friends, family, and even ourselves, better. *If only we weren't so drained!* We may even know the need for self-care, but it just seems too complicated and time-consuming.

Can we continue on like this? Our lives *seem* fine – even great – from the outside. We have a lot to be thankful for.

But life can be so exhausting! We know we need to make a change NOW, before we end up losing our health, relationships, and quality of life!

Just ask me. I know this one.

As an athlete, I learned to play through injuries to get the prize, at the expense of my body. As an adult, I tended to take on more and more, at the expense of my sanity. As a mom, I constantly multitasked to get it all done, at the expense of connecting to Joy, and modeling that for my children.

I received wake-up calls along the way, repeatedly. I remember vividly the physical messages that warned me to get out of the "Do Do" mindset. On the first day of a sport tryout camp, I knew I had hurt my shoulder, but the prize for succeeding was a trip to Rio de Janeiro to compete in a world championship. Come on! There was no way I was going to whine about a boo-boo in my shoulder! So I played on.

It was years later that I discovered my shoulder had been separated. Talk about being disconnected!

Fast forward two decades. I was with a doctor looking at x-rays of my neck. "So when did you break your neck?" she asked. Shocked, I told her point blank, "Never." Eventually, I realized that in a collision YEARS before, I had broken two vertebrae in a Sunday-morning fun-soccer-league for men and women over forty. Once again, I was so disconnected that I didn't even realize the pain I had been in for so long, let alone that I was so close to spinal cord damage!

Finally, I listened; I got the message, and recognized that I absolutely had to change my path, and although it took awhile, I learned to exercise my mind and body in a way to reconnect with the Joy of living!

I decided to become a personal trainer to help women build and recover healthy bodies. Over the years I have encountered too many stories of unintentional self-neglect. So many women put the needs of their jobs, and especially loved ones, ahead of their own needs. They have an inkling that something must be done to keep from losing themselves, but rescuing their health and happiness can be overwhelming! Who has time? Where does one even start?

What if, we could simplify the process of caring for ourselves, and keep that mind, body and Spirit connection? What if we could build these skills into our regular fitness routines and practice them consistently so they become easy to bring into everyday life? Thanks to the injuries I suffered due to being so disconnected, I have learned many of these skills and now practice them within my health and fitness regimen.

I call them the BALANCE Basics. They have become part of my daily life and have greatly strengthened my mind and body connection to Joy. If this path can help anyone uphold their quality of life, I am happy to share. Each letter in BALANCE represents a step toward inner and outer fitness and strengthening the connection of mind, body and Spirit. I have included some tips and examples of how I practice many of these steps in my small group fitness workouts.

THE B A L A N C E BASICS TO FLEX YOUR JOY

B – is for Breathe!!!!

Engaging in daily-focused breathing practices, even just for a minute or two at a time, will cleanse tension and resistance from mind and body and improve the ability to deal with specific challenging situations and life in general. Conscious breathing provides health and healing to the mind and body on many levels and allows access to our Spirit.

Try a simple "cleansing breath" exercise. Stop what you're doing, and take a long, slow breath through your nose. Feel the breath fill your belly, lungs and chest. Hold it for a second or two, and exhale long and slow through the nose. Empty the air from your lungs, chest, then belly. Exhale all tension from the body and the mind, and all the air from the belly. After at least two more of these breaths, take notice of how your body feels. More relaxed? Calm? Grounded? Do this anytime you need to regroup.

**I use this or another short breathing exercise with my groups at the beginning and the end of every workout session.*

A – Align

Align your thoughts and actions with your heart.

There are positive emotions that stem from love and Joy, and negative emotions that stem from fear. Once you have the ability to identify a negative emotion and recognize that it may not serve you, you are free to change your thoughts to make them positive. This may require time and help, but well worth the effort! When your thoughts are positive and aligned with your actions in what you wish to achieve, you know you are on the right path to your goal and it will be a smoother journey.

For fitness, select the exercises *and thoughts* that are beneficial to getting the results you want. For instance, if you are working on healing a bad back and doing a rehabilitative exercise, tell yourself "I feel this movement is slowly working my back muscles and making them strong." This is more beneficial than, "I hate this stupid, slow, boring exercise!"

***After the opening breathing exercise, I often verbalize an intention, such as "Feel the cells of your body smile as we honor them. Enjoy everything you experience in the next hour. Let go of tension and unnecessary thoughts."**

L – Let Go!

Let go of what does not benefit you.

In real life, this can refer to releasing both emotional and physical clutter. There are many tools to help us let go of unnecessary beliefs and thoughts. Journaling is a common means of unburdening ourselves of thoughts by writing them down. Expressing gratitude in any way is one of the best ways to let go of negative thinking and emotion.

In exercise, letting go can refer to old routines and exercises that no longer serve our needs. For me, it was impact sports that jarred my badly-aligned neck and put me at risk for deeper injury.

It can also refer to letting go of unnecessary tension in the body, negative thinking and other non-relevant thoughts. For example, release the muscles of the neck or jaw, when working arms or legs. Keep your mind in the moment, and focused on your movements to make them more efficient and beneficial. Release thoughts of worry about what's for dinner or even bigger problems. *No amount of "worry" has ever helped any situation!*

**In exercise as in life, look for opportunities to laugh. Laughter, the best medicine, allows us to let go of everything. Work out with someone you can laugh with!*

A – Activity!

Your mind *and* body need activity.

Keep your mind healthy through mental activities like mastering a new language, and solving problems or puzzles such as Sudoku.

Keep your body healthy by engaging in regular movement that increases heart rate, resistance exercise that strengthens muscles, and stretching to maintain flexibility and release tension.

Remember to choose enjoyable workout routines that help you Flex Your Joy. Repeatedly completing workouts that you dislike where you flex your stress, can actually aggravate your health!

**Find physical activities that you enjoy that keep your mind positive AND work your body. Workout with a friend or group of friends! Most of my clients come to me for general fitness and FUN, so we rev up metabolism, and build strength, stamina, and ...flexibility. They enjoy the weight loss, stress relief and more defined bodies resulting from the full mind/body workout and LOVE that we keep the mind positive. By socially interacting throughout, using music, dance moves, and variety, the activities are fun and the time passes quickly.*

N – Nutrition!

Feed your cells what they need to thrive!

Eat close to the earth. That means plenty of fruits and vegetables as they provide many required nutrients, hydration, and are full of antioxidants to help neutralize free radicals! Stick to *whole grains*, and *healthy* fats and proteins. Limit processed sugars and "white trash"...white rice, white flour, white potatoes, and other carbs devoid of nutrients.

And take high quality nutritional supplements! The jury is no longer out. There is no doubt that almost everyone can benefit from nutritional supplementation. The Surgeon General even stated years ago that taking a multi-vitamin is wise. Do the research and purchase products that have been well tested and proven by experts. A quality multivitamin should provide the levels of vitamins and minerals to help lower the risk of the major diseases that plague our society – like cancer, heart disease, stroke, and diabetes. Remember, you get what you pay for.

**Take your multivitamins daily. Before, during and after exercise, hydrate the cells with clean, purified water.*

C – Calm your cells!

Our body is made up of trillions of cells that serve as our foundation. Any structure will crumble if the foundation is not strong.

Cells are aggravated by toxins that destroy them. Toxins enter our bodies through the air we breathe, the water we drink, the food we eat, what we touch and what we put on our skin. They create free-radicals that can lead to inflammation, which is now known to cause or exacerbate not only achy joints and aging, but also more than 85% of diseases known to man, including many cancers!

Practice avoiding toxins by limiting excess sun exposure, cigarette smoke, unfiltered water, pesticides and preservatives in food, as well as in cleaning and skin-care products. In doing this, we can make a difference in how we feel, look *and* age!

Getting at least seven hours of uninterrupted, peaceful sleep daily provides cells with longer periods of time to be calm, so they can thrive, repair and heal. In addition, take daily breaks of focused breathing, prayer and meditation.

**Incorporate Yoga moves and breathing to bring stillness into your fitness routine. I like to end my sessions with Shavasana, or Corpse Pose, where we lie down, and breathe into total relaxation and stillness. We become aware of how it feels to be so calm that real healing and renewal takes place effortlessly. Remember this wonderful, relaxed feeling in other moments of the day.*

E – Elationships!

Build *Elationships.*

I first heard this word at a workshop from a gentleman quoting his friend Simone. Simone says an *Elationship* is a relationship without the "R" for resistance. I love this word and definition!

Nurture your Elationship with your higher power.

It is *vital* to create an *Elationship* with yourself, and love yourself without resistance! Treat YOURSELF as well as you treat others you love.

Build *Elationships* with other people. Surround yourself with people who love you, support you, or at least make you feel good when you are around them. Avoid or limit time with people who bring you down and de-value you. If you must be around these people, find ways to care for yourself within this situation. A support group or counselor could be of help if required.

**I promote fun and friendship in my fitness sessions. Enjoying physical activities with friends and loved ones offers great opportunities to build elationships with others as well as supports the elationship you have with yourself. Live, love and laugh with yourself and others every day!*

Our mind produces our thoughts. Our body generates our actions. Our Spirit guides us with emotions. Today's hectic lifestyle tends to interfere with the collaboration between mind, body and Spirit. When we take time to **B**reathe deeply, **A**lign with our hearts, **L**et go of what does not serve us, stay **A**ctive, have healthy **N**utrition practices, allow time for regenerating **C**alm, and build **E**lationships, we are best able to maintain that vital mind, body and Spirit connection. From here, we are closer to leading the lives of Joy that we were meant to live!

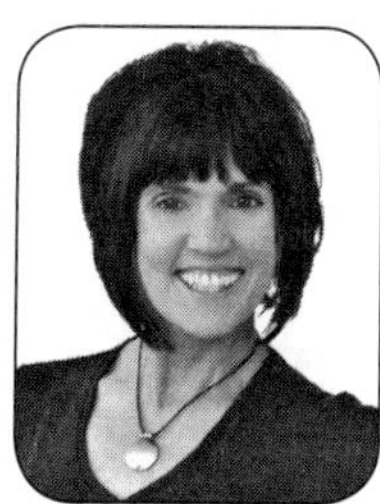

About Dorothy

Dorothy Jantzen is the owner of *Flex Your Joy* in Pleasanton, California where she is certified as a Personal Trainer and Wellness and Nutrition Consultant, and is a Yoga instructor in training. She specializes in Fitness, Friends and Fun small group classes, and promotes joy in exercising and exercising for Joy. She grew up in Canada and has a Bachelor of Physical Education degree from the University of British Columbia.

Dorothy accidently concentrated years of study as a patient in sports medicine due to having been a competitive athlete and earning numerous sports injuries. This personal rehabilitation education served her well when she became a Personal Fitness Trainer in the 90's – often using her great expertise in injury recovery. At this point she began a deeper study of nutrition, and through applying this knowledge to herself she suffered a serious outbreak of incredibly good health. She quickly became a disciple of natural healing and spent time in programs at the Chopra Center for Wellbeing and the Optimum Health Institute among others. Continuing her quest to heal old sports injuries, she experienced everything from physical therapy, Homeopathy, Naturopathy, Acupuncture, Rolfing, micro-current therapies, many bodywork therapies, Yoga and Pilates to a variety of spiritual healing practices.

Dorothy has kept her sense of humor throughout everything and knows her work is to lead other women to inner and outer fitness, and get back to having fun in life.

To learn more and receive a free "Time to Breathe" mini-relaxation audio, visit: www.FlexYourJoy.com

CHAPTER 25

The New Warrior Blueprint for Health & Longevity

By Sincere Hogan

Although on an individual level, the majority of us have different goals and reasons for those goals, in terms of diet and exercise. However, collectively, I am willing to bet we share one common goal: to live fuller, richer, and healthier lives. I mean, let's think about it, does anyone truly wake up and say, "Today, I want to feel miserable, be more stressed out, and totally feel like I don't want to get through this day. In fact, once I do, I will do it again, tomorrow." I doubt it.

Let's face it, due to life's everyday stresses and a constant need to multitask; it may appear as though we are constantly losing in a daily war of attrition. However, the road to true health and longevity is not traveled by survivors. It's conquered by warriors... New Warriors.

In order to be the New Warrior of today, we must approach the battles of life with the right weapons. Although each of our personal stresses may seem complicated, we can begin to overcome those stresses with simple approaches. The key word here is "simple." Attempting to overcome all of life's many stresses, simultaneously, is a losing battle. However, in order to overcome one big war on stress, you must begin by achieving victory one small battle at a time.

By the way, I'm going to let you in on a little secret. No matter how much you attempt to adjust your eating habits, or take on a fitness regimen, both will often seem unachievable and daunting, when you add both to other stresses you are most likely facing. Unfortunately, compared to the juggling act of work, family, and paying the bills, keeping your diet in check and penciling in daily physical activity become highly expendable.

Although you may have heard the phrase, "you have to make time for yourself," rarely are there any simple and actionable steps offered after the previous statement is made. However, I'm here to share the following blueprint of health and longevity for today's New Warrior, along with easy-to-apply components. These extremely doable tips will help you begin to take on and win the war on stress, regain that much-needed balance in your life, as well as open the doors to enjoying a healthier diet and fitness program.

I. MOVING TO THE GROOVE OF LONGEVITY

The key to making any health and fitness program work for you, is to find and do the program that works specifically for you. There is so much information on how you can be healthier, stronger, fitter, slimmer, etc., that it can often feel like you're experiencing information overload. The one issue that most of these providers of info for your health have is that the majority of these "experts," especially those involved in mainstream media, do not have a clue about who you are, your health background, your genetic makeup, your stress levels, your schedule, or other information needed to begin to truly create a health and fitness program designed specifically for you, the individual. Most programs on diet and fitness, shared by mainstream media, are pretty much general information or "cookie-cutter" at best.

The first step you should make, in order to find the wellness program that works specifically for you, is the program you dictate on your own terms. Now, don't get me wrong. I'm not saying just start doing any and every fitness program or fad diet known to man. Every great victory begins with a plan, once you have your specific goal in mind. You may have heard that you should begin your plans with the end in mind. However, in terms of health and longevity, it's obvious what "the end" is. Focusing 100% with the end in mind, in this case, can spark a sense of negativity and fear. Thus, instead of putting a health and fitness plan into place that promotes an active strategy for longevity, a reactive and stagnant plan to avoid a future that you have no clue of how it will happen, keeps you from taking control of your health right here, right now.

As I previously stated, in order to be today's New Warrior, we must approach the battles of life with the right weapons. The key word here is "approach." In other words, we have to be in the moment or as I like to put it, moving to our groove. Life is about movement. Looking closely at the word "movement," you can find the background to the groove of life: "We were meant to move!" However, there is no set rule that says we were meant to move 5-8 reps (steps) at a time for 5 sets (events) at a time. There are also no rules that say movement must be confined to a gym, 3 days a week, for 12 weeks only. We have to get moving and keep moving (with purpose), in order to feel alive. Yet, in order to fully enjoy that feeling, you must move on "your" personal terms, for "your" specific reasons, and not the reasons the evening news, the fitness magazines, or those creepy internet ads that appear mysteriously while you're checking your email, tell you.

Here are some great suggestions to consider, when planning or seeking help with the design of your personal physical fitness program:

1. **Make your plan work for you, and not you working for it.** It's time to stop trying to be the "perfectly healthy" person described in fitness and lifestyle magazines, talk

shows, and the evening news. The first step to consider, before embarking on your journey, is to check with your medical professional. Your medical professional can give you a more personalized idea of where you need to start.

2. **The best time to train or include physical activity, is the time you schedule to do so.** Make a daily appointment to get up and get moving, at least for 30 minutes a day. If you think you don't have time, take a look at your current daily activities. Consider trading in some email checking, social media engaging, and/or TV time for some get-up-and-go time! Trust me, the email will still be there, and I doubt someone will delete you from their friends list, if you're M.I.A. for 30 minutes. Oh, as for the TV, get a DVR in your life, set it, and get going.

3. **Be flexible.** Being physical doesn't mean you have to be confined to a gym. One of the best gyms in the world, and my personal favorite, is almost always accessible and free….the great outdoors.

4. **Partner Up!** Starting a fitness program doesn't have to be a lonely journey. Power is in numbers. In this case, why not invite a friend, family, or co-worker, with similar goals, to join you on your fitness journey? Studies have shown people are more likely to stick with a fitness or diet program, when they have accountability partners. If you have trouble finding an accountability partner offline, why not go "online." Various social media outlets, such as Facebook, Twitter, and various online forums are readily accessible, and make finding an accountability partner for your health and fitness journey as easy as typing in a website address.

5. **Be Specific.** Know exactly what it is that you want to accomplish. This is called, "Knowing Your *Why*." Simply stating, "I need to lose weight because I'm fat," or "I need to get rid of this gut" is simply not enough to motivate

you to keep going, when taking on your new program seems too difficult to continue. The desire to be alive and healthy enough to see your children graduate, the need to break the family-related pattern of suffering from diabetes before you're 40, or getting a grasp on your health in order to avoid the threat of heart disease before age 50, like all of the men in your family, is a lot more specific and a lot more motivating to continue the course of your daily health and fitness lifestyle.

These are just a small set of tips to get you going. However, each one is very doable. The most important thing to remember is that, as humans, we were made to move. Yet, moving frequently should not be a daunting task. It should be natural, enjoyable, and meaningful. Therefore, the first step to moving to your own groove towards longevity is to move to the beat of your own drum. Do what works for you, because you can only be the best "you" that you can be.

II. THE 3 STEPS TO RECOVER, REBUILD, & RELEASE STRESS

Throughout my years as a fitness professional, I've discovered that for every person who finds participating in a daily physical fitness program as challenging as finding Big Foot, there is another one who cannot go a day without some sort of physical activity. Come on, we all know "that" person. They are the ones who spend 2-3 hours in the gym each day. They are the ones who reverently proclaim "they must workout or train every day, or they will get depressed." They are the ones whose closet is probably filled with 25 colors of the same jogging outfit.

Don't get me wrong. I'm all for performing some sort of physical activity on a daily basis. However, my personal mantra that I share with all of my clients is: "For as many minutes as you train or are active, you must spend at least the same number of minutes recovering." In other words, if you spend 30 minutes being active and breaking a sweat, be sure to set aside another 30 minutes to relax, recover, restore, and rebuild.

The road to better health and longevity is all about balance. How you recover, in contrast to your physical activity, is no exception. However, recovery is not limited to just being a complement to physical activity. Recovery is a complement to the everyday stresses of life, such as work, home life, unexpected stress-related or traumatic events, emotional stress, and even our favorite stress…traffic. Well, it may not be our favorite. However, utilizing the following three tips will make dealing with traffic and the other previously mentioned stress-related events a lot less… well, …"stressful."

1. **Just Breathe.** We cannot live without breathing. As a matter of fact, there is more truth to that statement than we may realize. In stressful situations, if we take a moment to breathe, we may find that we've given ourselves time to let the stressful situation pass, or at least given us time to develop an appropriate response to the stress. Although breathing, in theory, is an involuntary response to life, there are ways to make it a voluntary response, as well. In order to better deal with stressful situations, we have to practice making breathing a voluntarily response tool for health and longevity. Here is a great exercise you can perform anywhere and anytime:

   a. Find a quiet place free of distractions (my favorite is the bathroom or the terrace).

   b. Sit tall, with legs close together and your hands flat on your thighs.

   c. Close your eyes.

   d. Listen and focus on your breathing.

   e. Inhale slowly for 8 counts.

   f. Hold your breath for 1 second.

   g. Slowly exhale for 6-8 counts.

   h. Repeat.

You can perform this breathing exercise for as long as you need. I like to do this exercise multiple times a day, for about 5 minutes. I find that once I perform this exercise, I am re-energized and ready to take on whatever tasks that await me. Also, by making this exercise a part of your daily routine, you may find you are a lot less reactive to stressful situations. Consequently, you become a lot more responsive and in a position to make better decisions. Now that's what 'walking to the beat of your own drum' is all about.

2. **Disconnect In Order to Reconnect.** These days, we are more connected than ever, thanks to various aspects of the internet, including: email, social media websites, online gaming, Skype, as well as on-demand streaming of movies and TV. Let's not forget how connected we are via our mobile phones. Not only do we have the capabilities to reach out and call just about anyone, anywhere, but due to accessibility of the web via our mobile phones, all of the aforementioned internet connectivity is no longer limited to our computers. We can take all of this connectivity with us, on the go.

   However, despite all of the technological advances in connectivity, the one aspect of staying connected seems to be slowly becoming a thing of the past – getting out and spending time with real people, in the real world. As human beings, we are hardwired to want to connect and be in the presence of others. Instead of sending a text or email to an old friend, why not meet up for coffee, lunch, or a walk in the park, and catch up? Even if friends are far away, you can connect and meet new like-minded friends via websites such as Meetup.com, church, or after-work events, just to name a few. Here's a fun challenge. Why not simply start a conversation with a complete stranger, today? You never know what you may learn, or how great you will make someone feel, by showing interest in them, including yourself.

3. Give More in Order to Get More. In my opinion, there is nothing more fulfilling than giving. I've always believed the more you give, the more blessings you receive. I'm not saying to give with the expectation of receiving something in return. Give for the sake of giving, especially to those who could benefit from the blessings you can share. The rest will take care of itself. The most important gift you receive in return is how good it feels to reach out and help someone. I think it's pretty safe to say that, if you feel good, then there's no room for stress; thus, there's now more room for being healthy.

Often, the art of giving is compartmentalized to monetary giving. However, here is a list of the many ways you can give and enrich the lives of others, as well as enrich the life of your own:

- Volunteer at a local homeless shelter
- Volunteer to read to an elementary school class
- Mentor a teen
- Volunteer at your local animal shelter
- Provide transportation to the elderly to the grocery store, to run errands, to vote, or offer to take care of their errands and pick up their groceries for those that are sick and shut-in
- Donate clothing to your local homeless or women's shelter
- Coordinate fundraisers for your favorite charity
- and so much more…

The possibilities are endless. Most importantly, you are doing good and feeling good at the same time. By implementing the art of giving, as well as any or all of the tools I have provided in this blueprint for health and longevity, you will find that life becomes more enjoyable and less stressful. In fact, you will feel so good that you could take on the world with a smile. That's what traveling the road to a healthier life and increasing your chances for longevity is all about. As a matter of fact, that's what being today's New Warrior is all about, as well.

- Eat like a warrior

- Train like a warrior

- "Live" like a warrior

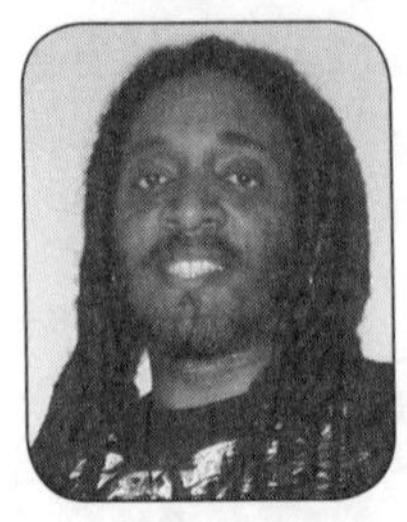

About Sincere

Sincere Hogan is the owner of New Warrior Media and the creator of New Warrior Training Systems, based in Houston, TX. Better known as "The People's Fit Coach" Sincere's mission is to coach, empower, and inspire individuals to tap into their varied resources, in order to create the health and fitness lifestyle they truly desire.

For nearly a decade, Sincere's New Warrior Training Systems' holistic blend of mental programming, training recovery, bodyweight, kettlebell, and unconventional training methods has successfully helped countless clients of various age groups, fitness ranges, and backgrounds, exceed their goals and expectations. Sincere is truly a connoisseur of the art of human movement, and loves to share that passion with others, at every available opportunity.

Sincere is the author of the best-selling *Ultimate Bodyweight Conditioning for Strength & Fat Loss* DVD. He has successfully coached 12 teams, in preparation for the Men's Health **URBANATHLON®** annual race in Chicago (2009 & 2010), and has been featured regularly on numerous television and radio stations, and has been interviewed, featured, and contributed fitness articles in nationally-published magazines and newspapers such as: *Family Energy, IronMan Japan, Family Digest, My Mad Methods, The San Antonio Express News, Health & Fitness Sports Magazine* and various health and fitness sites on the web.

Sincere has been featured regularly on Houston's Fox 26 Morning News "Workout Wednesdays," and was also featured as the exclusive trainer for Clear Channel Radio's Arrow 93.7's "World's Biggest Loser" contest. Sincere has also been featured on more than one occasion on radio stations.

Hogan, is a proud father and husband, and currently lives in Texas with his beautiful wife, Paulette.

To learn more about Sincere Hogan, "The People's Fit Coach," or to join his New Warrior Nation newsletter, filled with healthy recipes, training tips and videos, and more, visit: http://newwarriortraining.com.

CHAPTER 26

Creating a Road Map to Health, Wellness and Balance

By Doug Duerr

Is it time to take inventory? In business we must take a good look at what works and what does not work to be successful. Many times we are faced with the decision to let go of products, services and sometimes people, that do not serve our business and add value to its success. This is one of many learning tools that we may need to use and apply in our own lives.

We all must take an inventory of our life and face the truth so that we can move forward with greater ease and success.

If life thus far has presented a series of challenges, remember you are not alone. They have been seasons of temporary circumstances. If you feel you've had a bit longer than a normal season of challenges, I might suggest we begin by removing any victim-consciousness statements.

In my own personal life and professional experience I have found a pathway to finding that illusive creature we call "balance." Being out of balance affects all aspects of our life – our relationships, weight, health, emotional stresses, diet, business, and ultimately the way we perform in life. This also collectively affects our world. Did you know your responsibility is much larger than just you? OK, now I've given you another big burden to bear.

I understand. I spent more than half my life weaving through stages of what I refer to as "victimhood." Did I have good reason? Well, don't we all?

I discovered a method of healing while acknowledging my back story, but choosing not to live in it; declutching from the trappings of a vicious cycle of "victimhood" and honestly releasing and writing a new story to a brilliant future! Then, I was able to become a vessel that could help others find their own level of balance and success. My coaching practice was born!

Several years ago my mission statement was written:

Guiding people to create life balance through personal alignment and accountability. Claiming the "Today is Mine" principle.

This sounded great! It became my statement. Now, I had to put my statement into an action plan – beginning with me on my journey, with self-work to do, long before I could reach out and offer guidance to others.

I find in my coaching practice, brave, well-intended people making decisions to "get healthy," but they don't know what "healthy" looks like. Health is often associated with an external body image. Perhaps from mass media or a former image of a body type from their past. Rushing to a gym, starting some cardio, trying to "eat healthier," but the reality is most are lost. Jumping in blindly without a proper "mind-set" can quickly lead to failure. There must be a plan of action involving *all* of you. This is not just a body image. Your Mind, Body and Spirit must come into alignment and work together for success. Here's where we begin creating a road map to health and wellness in the direct path of life balance.

What is balance and how can I get there?

Most are searching for freedom from something. Starting with what they think they no longer want without giving consideration to what contributed to their journey so far.

When we recognize this and acknowledge the journey, a shift begins. A shift in thinking about ourselves. We become open and receptive and begin to set up our new belief system.

SETTING UP YOUR BELIEF SYSTEM

Let's Talk MIND: The pre-game work is most important! Your pre-game practice will set you up for optimal success!

This is your choice and commitment to action. Remember my mission statement? Create your statement. Write it out. This involves personal goals. Remember to write a positive statement in your written words. Remove "try's" and replace with "will's" and "do's." Write it and post it! State it everyday. Train your thinking to what you want your life to be. Health and Wellness? Financial freedom? An exit strategy from your job? Losing weight? What is it?

Total wellness in every aspect of life includes freedom from stresses over health and finances. Freedom from "worry bondage." This may be your goal. It is for most.

Let's begin by replacing old embedded toxic talk we've been telling ourselves for years. This self-sabotaging chatter holds us back from the good we know to clearly be ours. We begin our freedom and love ourselves more than the old stories. When we start to love ourselves and become the first priority, this is when we can truly take care of ourselves and then others.

You must come first!

WORDS ARE POWERFUL!

This clear and concise action step will assist you in manifesting the goals you set for your life.

This is the beginning of declutching from toxic chatter and limiting words and is where we find our next tool.

1. Remove "try" from your vocabulary. "Try" is a maybe. It is not clear.
2. Remove "I wish" or "I hope" and re-state it into "I believe."
3. Make your intentions known. Be Concise.
4. Be in agreement with your plan.
5. Tell the Truth to your heart. See your intentions as real and authentic.

TOOLS FOR THE TOOL BOX

In writing your statements and goals, you will find there may be a steady stream of thoughts and phrases that do not support you.

Ask yourself if the thought is creating a limitation in your life. I am sure there are many. They pop up during our training all the time. This is why it's a process to re-train your thinking.

"RE-BOOT BOOTCAMP" FOR THE MIND

Some thoughts come in to hold you back and limit you and need to be released. Are you ready? Not everyone is ready, this is why getting healthy and finding balance becomes a challenge for some.

Living in an impatient society we want "quick fixes." We prefer to skip steps and go directly to the finish line. This is not a race. It is your long, healthy, prosperous life. So, let's slow down and give this careful attention.

A release can be a difficult process. Be gentle with yourself. This exercise involves denials and affirmations. The D&A process may be new to you. Most understand an affirmation, but the power of the denial is often skipped.

For this example we'll use unwanted pounds as the challenge.

We often develop a hatred of something we no longer want in our lives, but carrying the hate, or dislike is far worse than extra body weight.

1. **<u>The Denial:</u>**
   "This extra weight (the actual number) I have carried for the last ten years no longer serves me. I understand it has served a purpose in my life. It has protected and served me for reasons I may not understand. Though I am grateful, I am now fully prepared to release this (the actual number) extra weight and the limitation it places on my life. Thank you and good bye."

2. **<u>The Affirmation:</u>**
   "My body is completely healthy and whole in all ways with no unnecessary extra weight to carry. I embrace my body; my life and a healthier me."

3. **<u>Gratitude:</u>**
   "I am grateful and I clearly see the steps I will take for my life to be successful, healthy and whole."

Always follow up the process with heartfelt gratitude. This informs our Mind, Body and Spirit to be in an awareness of the action we are taking. Congratulations! This is an action step! Long before your attempt to enter a gym or find the perfect food. **You are healing your mind and setting yourself up for Success!**

Now we have an agreement and are clear about the D&A. Remember, this is not denying the challenge or issue exists, it is denying that the condition, challenge or issue has power in your life.

We must stop giving away our power to conditions that are unfavorable or destructive to our well-being.

DECLUTTERING YOUR MIND.

It's much like an overfilled closet or garage. You can't bring in the new unless you get rid of the old clutter. It's time to release and let go! Again, we're talking about mind work, this also comes into action when we move into healthy nutrition and fitness.

This is a vital part of the success process to total health and well-being. We know the mind is an incredible tool, it is the beginning of your success transformation. It is the choices you make that lead to your successes.

There are foods, tonics, lotions, supplements, juices and prayers that work well to assist you in accomplishing goals, but you still have work to do. You are a part of the process. It is in your attitude, mind-set, belief system and ultimately your choices.

When moving into nutrition we also start with our mind and belief system. It's also a trust factor in the person(s) that coach(es) and guide(s) you in the beginning.

Ask yourself questions:

1. Do you believe in the product or system?
2. Do you believe in your coach or trainer?
3. Most of all; Do you believe and trust in yourself?

If you find yourself in an "I don't know" or "I'm not sure" place, it's time to spend some time back on step one. The Mind. If you're not ready, be honest. Chances are, in some way, you have told yourself a few lies to mask the reality or come up with excuses along the way. Check yourself and get honest about your plan.

"Choices. You have the power to choose. Creating a space for good choices is an action step. Small steps build into large rewards. Take that small step with good intentions toward your own well-being and everyone will benefit as your choices ripple out to all of us."

~ Doug Duerr

THE BODY TEMPLE

When you begin to seek nutrition to feed your body, you want to stay close to the good earth. What is good earth today? Over the years, unfortunately we have changed our earth and the way we produce our fruits, vegetables and our healthy proteins.

With the progression of big business and greed we have allowed the use of pesticides and toxic chemicals intended for disease-free crops and fast growth, but we have depleted our good earth from vital minerals and nutrients needed for healthy human and animal consumption.

So what do we do now? There are answers and it can be found on my bio page and web site - The Nutrition Key. I spent several years searching out only the best for my body, my family and clients – eliminating stress over what to eat and where to find highly nutritional food and supplements. After much research, I discovered an ethically sound company and I no longer have worry or concern about perfect nutrition. A Blessing? Yes!

Remember, when you are making nutritional decisions; here is some "food for thought" in your planning:

1. Where is this product coming from and it's source?
2. If it's animal or vegetable, what did it consume or was treated with before it came in contact with my body temple?

TIME TO GET MOVIN'

In as little as 28 days! A short amount of time to reverse years of negative or unhealthy behaviors and toxicity. You are feeling great inside and feeding your mind and body optimal nourishment with your words and nutrition. Now, we can get movin' with the fitness!

Cardiovascular fitness is a requirement in our lives!

Some health seekers go out and hit it hard and eventually fail due to the excuses and the "toxic talk." This time, for you, it is different.

We began with re-booting the mind, making clear statements about what we're seeking and we are taking action steps to write down our mission and read it everyday.

We spend time on releasing and letting go of embedded thoughts and behaviors.

Using our tools of denials and re-enforcing new choices with affirmations and remembering our gratitude. We began feeding our body with good balanced optimal nutrition.

We now begin to feel so much more alive, the enthusiasm and energy of what we are feeding our mind and body kicks in. We are eager to get moving.

A brisk walk may become a jog and a dance may become a party of self discovery. Group exercise classes are an excellent way to add connections with like minded people and offer a variety of fitness levels. Be open to discovering all the ways and methods you can increase your heart rate. You will find encouragement by surrounding yourself with those that support your new lifestyle.

Exercise may vary depending on your current level, age and abilities at this point. You'll want to check with your health care professional to be certain you have no current restrictions. Some days you may only have the time for 30 minutes while others you can go longer. Start logging your miles. Set, achieve and increase your goals. Remember, there are no more obstacles between you and your health. You come first. Your total health and wellness are priority One.

You are now aware of the formula and the plan for your re-boot boot camp. Are you ready?

HEALTHY SPIRIT

In the Mind, Body and Spirit approach to health and well-being, where does the healthy Spirit kick in?

Your Spirit, your very wise and healthy higher Self is, and always has been, completely healthy. It is your Spirit that is always there. It is that brilliant, motivating, loving part of you that has been the voice that knows clearly what to do. Some call it a "still small voice within" while others call it "intuition," and on some level people refer to it as "a higher power," "Universe" or "God."

Our Higher Self, our Spirit within is always healthy, honest and authentic. We choose sometimes to not listen and hear what we truly need to do and be in our lives. We often allow the chatter and ego to get in the way and try to silence our Spirit. We may think it is not there at times, but when we still our minds and listen we hear the clear answers. Your Spirit is healthy and whole. It is complete and desires only to be your true guide and coach. Once you have listened and allow your Spirit to lead, you may no longer need to seek outside yourself. Once you have put your words and belief system into action and fed your mind and body, your Spirit will repay you greatly.

I trust and I believe the words, formula and tips we used in this chapter as we began to create your road map to health, wellness and balance will contribute to great successes in all aspects of your life. Healthy Abundant Living! Mind, Body and Spirit.

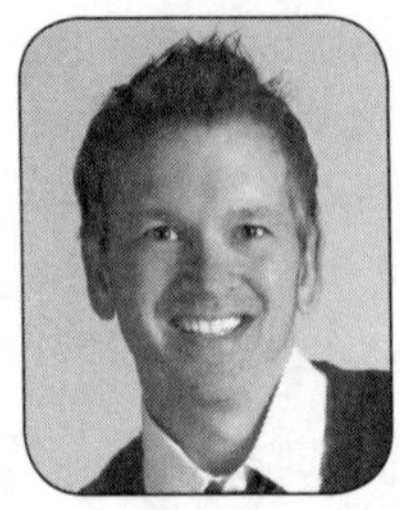

About Doug

Doug Duerr is a Healthy Living Life Coach, Author, Speaker and Yoga teacher. He also serves regularly with grief groups and in workshops throughout the year. Doug is a published author of *The Adventures of Jazz and Elliott,* a colorful series encouraging children the freedom to imagine and discover.

He is affiliated with the Y of Greater Houston, Unity of Houston, and N.E.S.T.A. As the owner and principle coach of MY LIFE Coaching based in Houston, TX, his wellness company stays active in training and education within their mission as an advocate for optimal wellness available to every person. A lifelong resident of Texas, Doug enjoys a variety of lifestyles and cultures, he easily adapts and finds joy in the piney woods, the beautiful hill country or is just as happy in the heart of Manhattan.

Doug has partnered with the world leader in nutrition; Isagenix International, the nutritional key to serve the many health and financial-minded individuals. This coach understands what it takes to live balance; reminding himself, his clients, and students daily, to be accountable and discover life. His hobby of latin dance is just one of many ways he acknowledges his Spirit and lives the example of his teachings. He has a deep appreciation and love for animals and is a rescue advocate.

Balance is a common goal for most students and clients. As a holistic planner focusing on wellness, Doug's approach is a lifestyle choice to Optimal Wellness and emphasizes the whole person. It is the integration of the body, mind, and Spirit; and the appreciation that everything we do, think, feel, and believe has an impact on our health. This is also what he adopts and delivers as a course to clients. "We have become more of a society about alleviating or curing a disease, this wellness approach encourages a personal responsibility for well-being."

This proactive and preventive action is designed to achieve optimum levels of health, social and emotional functioning. His personal practice encourages clients and groups to achieve this highly sought after goal.

Doug has discovered when a person is open and coachable to the tools, anyone can become empowered and create a shift in their life – creating wellness within relationships, fitness, finances, nutrition, career and spirituality – and ultimately the relationship with Self.

MY LIFE Coaching encourages a wellness-oriented lifestyle adopting habits and behaviors that promote wholeness. It involves the recognition that we all have physical, psychological, social, and spiritual needs, with each dimension necessary for life balance.

Live Life Now! Doug Duerr is a master guide, coach and trainer for the client or student that is coachable, ready for action and ultimately responsible for their wellness.

Visit: www.todayismine.net and
www.mylifecoaching.net

The Nutrition Key: www.dougduerr.isagenix.com

CHAPTER 27

Occupational Wellness!

By Raymond James

What is occupational wellness? What is the best way to go about achieving it? When it comes to wellness, some areas of your life may be more easily measured than others. Also, to what degree you are physically, emotionally, spiritually, intellectually, occupationally, relationally, or environmentally well is dependent on your perspective. However, it is imperative to be aware that all these elements of wellness are interdependent. Even with that, a recent global research poll revealed that career wellbeing is the leading element of wellness. For it is the work you do that will occupy the majority of your time. Interestingly, career wellbeing is not one of the aforementioned elements where life demands reflection, until you realize that it falls under occupational wellness.

Most people mistake career and occupational wellbeing as being synonymous, and by standard definition they are, until you realize that you have to consider everything that occupies your time. Occupy, by definition, is "to engage the attention or energies of." While I challenge you to pay very close attention to and dynamically balance all the details of your day that occupy your energies, here we will discuss how to go about finding what career(s) will provide you with the opportunity for satisfaction at work and in life.

Let's illustrate with a story about Joseph, who represents the more than half of working adults that are dissatisfied with their work. Joseph is not exactly sure how he ended up where he is and wants to make a change, take time off, and do whatever it takes to escape his current situation; if only he could. Most people think Joseph is happy because he has everything. He makes really good money, has a degree in business administration, is a high-level manager at an advertising company, and has the prospects of becoming an executive leader or maybe even the CEO someday. Joseph lives in a beautiful home in a great neighborhood. He is married to a terrific woman and is blessed with incredible, healthy children. As a matter of fact, Joseph has the appearance of a modern-day success story. Yet, even with all that, Joseph just isn't thriving and he isn't happy!

Back in high school, Joseph listened to what all the outside influences in his life told him: think about what he might want to do when he gets older, go to college to get an education, and then go to work to become happy and successful. There were no detailed instructions or much of a process to go through, so Joseph didn't really give it much thought. He just went about his studies and applied to college. As it turns out, he changed his major three times and it took him almost six years to get his four-year degree. He never even got a job with his accounting degree. He has been in sales and marketing his whole career. Well, he didn't realize that the decisions he made early in his life would affect his ability to be happy. He just thought work would make him the money he needed to be happy. He had absolutely no perspective or insight into what truly drives him. Even as he got older, as he met people with unique jobs and careers, he wondered "how come he never heard of that job before?" Since more than half of working adults are dissatisfied with their work, maybe you have imagined what it would be like to do certain work and said once or twice before, "...that you could see yourself enjoying that really cool job, had you only known."

Joseph's dissatisfaction and frustration continued to grow and was affecting everything at work, at home, with his social life, and especially his health. He lost his motivation to exercise which affected his energy level and he began packing on the pounds. No matter how hard he tried to leave his work frustrations behind, he always ended up taking it out on his family at home. Then, of course, at every social event the first question people ask is, "how is work going?" That just spoiled the rest of the event due to all the thoughts and emotions that encircled his job. He asked himself, "is this what the rest of his life was going to be like?" He just knew he had to do something before his dissatisfaction at work made things worse.

So he began to gather information and set out on a quest to find work he will love. He had no idea where to start but remembered taking assessments at work that told him his personality type and behavioral styles, but he didn't really understand what it meant to be (ENTP) extroverted, intuitive, thinking, perceiving. Then there was the other test that labeled him as dominant and influential, and not so steady or conscientious. Besides the results of each test were 25 pages of technical terms he didn't understand; he especially didn't appreciate being told he craved attention, wasn't reliable and that he had no feelings. Moreover, nobody at the company really understood how to apply any of it. They even told him not to worry about the assessments because it was just something the company's Human Resources department needed for the file. You see, companies know that personality types and behavioral styles are not indicators of future job performance. For an example, just look at Tom Cruise and Val Kilmer in the movie "Top Gun." Two distinctly different personalities yet they were the two best pilots in the Navy. You probably know people right now that are really good at the same job, and yet have distinctly different personalities and behavior styles.

As it turns out, corporations have been utilizing scientific instruments to qualify/ disqualify candidates and pigeonhole employees into certain positions for many years. Even with all these tools, employee engagement remains at historical lows. While several factors could play in to the low engagement numbers, the studies are still true that the majority of people are dissatisfied with their current line of work. Through the years, assessments have evolved to include more modern, holistic philosophies, but have yet to emerge as practical tools in the workplace. An entire industry is quickly gaining popularity in the field of career development that is outside of corporations and government-funded mandates. These programs are being sought out by adults looking to transition or are unemployed. Now even HS and college-age students are engaging in this more intuitive process hoping to avoid costly bad decisions, so as to head off the mid-life scramble that Joseph is in.

Certainly, Joseph was excited to now immerse himself in this intuitive process of discovery, to gain awareness about how to find work he will love. The process consisted of three major modules, with several subtopics filled with questions and activities to bring to light the answers Joseph was seeking. The major modules are Discovery, Exploration, and Tools.

Discovery was the first, most important part of the program. The process of discovery provided insight into his personal strengths, preferences, work values, motivated skills and also delivered new perspectives for Joseph to consider. These are perspectives that he can use for a lifetime to become more intuitive and aware as he continued to find his way on the path of his journey. This all helped Joseph uncover his hidden passions and an even more defined purpose for his work and life.

In module two, Exploration, Joseph used a survey that allowed him to connect what he just learned about himself, to careers he could be passionate about. The survey was easily understood due to its use of everyday language. What Joseph really learned was that exploring new opportunities included getting below the surface of the job/ title to the details. After all, it was not just another job Joseph was after. He learned its the functions of that job, where he could use his strengths, assert his values, and use his motivated skills that would increase his chances for satisfaction – things that really matter ...such as the daily tasks, the knowledge he could apply each day, and the type of work environment he would be comfortable in. The results of the survey even allowed Joseph to learn about the education/ training requirements, the salary expectations, and the future employment outlook for the careers. Joseph was able to scour through dozens of potential careers where he actually had transferrable skills that he could apply. He began to get really excited about the prospects of making the changes he was looking for. He now began to look at what it would take to make the transition, even if it meant taking some college level courses at night or obtaining specific training certificates so he could move on. One thing he acknowledged was that it was a process that was well worth his time and effort.

Module three of the program excited Joseph because it included tools to help him plan his transition. Joseph enthusiastically began to embrace the idea of being a lifelong learner, even though he thought he was done with education when he finished his bachelors program, some fifteen (15) years ago. His first reminder, one he heard many times over the years, was on the character traits and rituals of successful, happy people. The program also gave him a refresher and some new ideas about money matters. One thing for certain was that there would be some changes in the household finances, where he had to work with his family on making some short-term lifestyle adjustments. He would also need their patience and understanding as he worked two steps backwards to go three steps forward and beyond. The next powerful lesson Joseph learned was about his way with time. For example, while Joseph was thinking it was too late and he was too old for a change, it was brought to his attention that he may very well have another 50 or more years of life left. How would that be if he kept his current path? Did you know that when men that lived beyond ninety five (95) years of age were asked what it was about their life that they lived so long? They responded "I had fun doing the work I did!" And sure, Joseph has a calendar with meeting schedules and events, but the perspective he gained on the best ways for him to use time more effectively just added to the tool chest he already had. Communication issues are always in the way of getting things done. This component of the program really shed some new light on how Joseph viewed his relationships. This piece even included how giving more of yourself to benefit others results in more positive life experiences. Finally, the program put all the information together by teaching a model for decision-making that would help him stay on track and grow, called 4DFocus, which included a planning tool called FocalPoint Map Method. Joseph sure was glad he decided to explore this potential change and is really motivated to take the necessary steps to execute his plan.

Now you might say Joseph just needs to write a resume and start networking, but in reality, until he looks deep inside himself to understand what really drives him, he will probably just find himself in the same situation. Joseph must identify, quantify and speak definitively about what he wants. He should not make the change just for change's sake.

Throughout the transition process, Joseph learned many things about himself and the activities he should engage in to occupy his time. Contrary to conventional thinking, he learned that focusing on using his strengths was much better than working to develop his weaknesses. That's not to say that Joseph shouldn't understand what he needs to improve on, it is just that a global research poll revealed that people that use their strengths every day in their work are three (3x) times more likely to have an excellent quality of life. He also was pleasantly surprised that when a survey or activity reveals his preferences, it means it is just his innate approach to the environment and the world around him – not that he doesn't possess any other characteristics or can't see another point of view. Besides the many other revelations, Joseph especially appreciated gaining the understanding that being an extrovert does not mean he is always craving to be the center of attention. It was really reassuring that he is both an extrovert and an introvert, and that the degree of his participation in any situation had to do with his level of comfort in the environment, with the people around him, and especially his interest in the topic being discussed. Can you imagine a room full of computer programmers, generally labeled as introverts, when they get together to discuss emerging technologies? I bet it is safe to say that the conversation involves quite a bit of enthusiasm looking to take center stage. Are they all newly converted extroverts? Of course not!

In the end, while Joseph has many things to do in order to accomplish a meaningful transition to a new and satisfying career, he sees his current circumstances and the prospects of his future much more clearly. He has new focus, a renewed vigor, and thriving fervor. Furthermore, Joseph came to understand that the critical components of doing work you love are being aware of your personal strengths, understanding your preferences, work values and motivated skills. Joseph will even tell you that it all really starts with having the right perspective; one of love and gratitude, mercy and forgiveness. His new point of view has helped him feel free about choosing and carefully considering the work and activities he engages in, and while life continually challenges Joseph to apply this each day, he is happily on his way to occupational wellness!

Occupational Wellness References

Wellbeing, Rath and Harter, Gallup Press New York, NY 2010

Employee Engagement Report 2011, BlessingWhite, Inc. Princeton, NJ

(ENTP) is a reference to the widely used Meyers-Brigg Type Indicator developed by Isabel Briggs Myers and Katharine Briggs and is based on Carl Jung's theory of psychological types.

Dominant, Influential, Steady, Conscientious are references to the widely used DISC psychological inventories developed by John Geier and is based on the 1928 work of psychologist William Moulton Marston and the original behaviorist Walter V. Clarke and others.

Extrovert/ Introvert approach to the environment is based on the Personal Style Model developed by Consulting Resource Group International (CRG); Sumas, WA

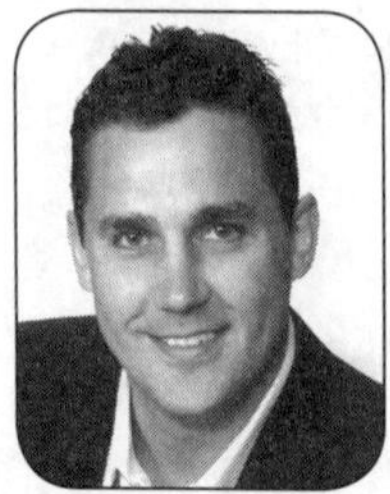

About Raymond

Raymond James, founder of Discovery Guidance Center, Certified Global Career Development Facilitator (GCDF), Certified Life Coach, NLP Practitioner. Raymond is sought after for his expert ability to lead clients on a path to reaching their full potential. As a career coach, Raymond embodies the leadership qualities needed to motivate students – to realize the dreams they have are well within their grasp. Developing people has always been the focus for Raymond, whether in the executive boardroom, at leadership development events, or even on the football field and the dojo.

Happiness and career success has many facets and unique meanings for every person. Raymond leads clients to discover new perspectives, allowing them to see the world through a new lens to slow the chaos and circumstances in which they feel stuck. Raymond's clients quantify their strengths, values, interests and motivations. They are able to see all the options they have, so they can make better choices.

Raymond is able to excite clients as they design new chapters in the story of their life. With these new crystal clear visions, clients learn to develop Focal Point Maps to carry out and deliver themselves in a more authentic way. The 4D Focus method is a tool that clients continue to use to adjust and grow as they move forward with their careers, and all the roles in their life.

To learn more about Raymond James and his Empowerment Programs, visit the Discovery Guidance Center at www.4Dguidance.net